More praise for *Misadventures of a Parenting Yogi*

"The potent blend of dad and yogi and humorist that Brian Leaf so deftly mixes makes his book a must-read for parents of any generation. I say namaste to a dad who can keep it light and lead with humor and stillness."
— Peggy O'Mara, founder of Mothering.com

"I found myself smiling, laughing, occasionally disagreeing, and, most important, thinking about where I stand as a parent. Brian Leaf's musings and misadventures come from the heart and encourage us to be on the parental dance floor while also consciously watching ourselves from the balcony."
— Kim John Payne, author of *Simplicity Parenting*, *Beyond Winning*, and *The Soul of Discipline*

"Fatherhood is not a spectator sport, and Brian Leaf isn't afraid to call the play-by-play on his own successes, near misses, and semi-disasters. He's funny and poignant, and gets across a powerful message about tuning in to our children and ourselves without proclaiming one right way to be a dad."
— Larry Cohen, author of *Playful Parenting*

"If parenting has as many laughs as this book, sign me up! Fans of the first *Misadventures* will delight in this romp through the trials, tribulations, messes, and joys of alternative child rearing — all captured with Leaf's trademark mix of humor, honesty, and compassion."
— Benjamin Lorr, author of *Hell-Bent: Obsession, Pain, and the Search for Something Like Transcendence in Competitive Yoga*

"Pattabhi Jois said that family life was the 'Seventh Series' of Ashtanga Yoga, the most challenging and almost impossible to perfect. If this warm, funny book — a love letter both to yoga and to his kids — is any indication, then Brian Leaf is a Seventh-Series Master."
— Neal Pollack, author of *Alternadad* and *Stretch*

"Brian Leaf writes about parenting and yoga with such humor that you almost forget how seriously important these topics are. His writing is a lighthearted reminder of how crucial humor, insight, and keeping things in perspective are to our children's and our own well-being. Brian reminds us to take our role as parents seriously but also to go ahead and have fun with it."

— Christy Turlington Burns, supermodel and founder of
Every Mother Counts

"Finally! A much-needed and elegant male perspective on parenting from a respected and respectful voice in the holistic community. Brian Leaf has struck the perfect balance between honesty, humor, passion, and compassion for all paths of parenting. What a wonderful addition to any parents' library; this is a wonderful gift to any expecting, recent, or seasoned mom or dad interested in conscious parenting, being truly present for their family, and finding the beauty in every challenge of being a caregiver."

— Mayim Bialik, PhD, actress on *The Big Bang Theory* and author of
Beyond the Sling

Misadventures *of a* PARENTING YOGI

Misadventures of a PARENTING YOGI

Cloth Diapers, Cosleeping, and My (Sometimes Successful) Quest for Conscious Parenting

Brian Leaf

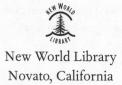

New World Library
Novato, California

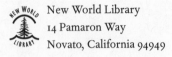

New World Library
14 Pamaron Way
Novato, California 94949

The material in this book is intended for education. It is not meant to take the place of diagnosis and treatment by a qualified medical practitioner or therapist. No expressed or implied guarantee of the effects of the use of the recommendations can be given or liability taken.

Text design by Tona Pearce Myers

Library of Congress Cataloging-in-Publication Data
Leaf, Brian.
Misadventures of a parenting yogi : cloth diapers, cosleeping, and my (sometimes successful) quest for conscious parenting / Brian Leaf.
    pages   cm
ISBN 978-1-60868-267-6 (pbk. : alk. paper) — ISBN 978-1-60868-268-3 (ebook)
1. Parenting. 2. Child rearing. 3. Parenthood—Humor. 4. Yogis. 5. Yoga. I. Title.
HQ755.8.L3746 2014
649'.1—dc23   2013049001

First printing, May 2014
ISBN 978-1-60868-267-6
Printed in Canada on 100% postconsumer-waste recycled paper

New World Library is proud to be a Gold Certified Environmentally Responsible Publisher. Publisher certification awarded by Green Press Initiative. www.greenpressinitiative.org

10 9 8 7 6 5 4 3 2 1

To Mom and Dad,
Swami Kripalu,
Noah and Benji,
and Gwen, of course

Parents live for the tiny vacations....
Like when you put your kids in the car and you close their door...
that little walk around to your own door?
It's like a Carnival Cruise.

— Louis C.K., *Chewed Up*

Contents

Author's Note

*A*ll opinions expressed in this work are mine and not those of my publisher (actually most are really my wife, Gwen's, but I accept them). All the events depicted actually happened, though at times I have tweaked the timeline to simplify the narrative. And all characters are real. Though I have often changed the names. For example, of Jeremiah. You can't complain about paying $400 for a person's poop-streaked cloth diapers and use his real name.

Preface

Lox 'n Latkes

I am a parent. I can prove it. Inside my coat pocket right now are one diaper (clean), one pair of children's underwear (soiled), one unscratched lottery ticket, and countless teething biscuit and rice cake crumbs.

I am also a yogi. Ten years ago, this was easier to prove. My pockets were filled with half-used class cards, a bookstore receipt for *Light on Yoga* or *The Ayurvedic Cookbook*, and folded-up handouts of Rumi and Kabir quotes. Now, ten years later, there's less time for yoga classes, and I'm reading parenting books instead of yoga books. But, still, my yoga is alive and well. My attempts at mindfulness and union are stronger than ever.

For example, this morning, after my family had breakfast at the Lone Wolf Café.

Noah, age six, loves the waffles, and I love the Lox 'n Latkes Benedict. After breakfast we are to drive a few miles to the Amherst winter farmers' market to shop and meet some friends. We finish breakfast and walk to the car, but Benji, age two, will not get into his car seat.

He is standing on the floor in the backseat and will not sit. To drive like this, with Benji not strapped in, is, of course, illegal and unsafe. So Gwen and I can't give in. We must get him buckled. Benji is crying and it's too cold outside to keep the windows open, so the noise in the car is building. Soon, very likely, in a domino effect, Noah will succumb to the noise and begin wailing in a cacophonous duet.

I have just read nineteen parenting books; surely I've got something up my sleeve.

I try Playful Parenting. "Benji, if you don't sit in that seat, well, I'm going to sing 'Yankee Doodle' until you do." I make a doofy expression and start singing.

No giggles. He's not buying it. He plants his feet onto the floor mat.

I try Simplicity Parenting. I relax my body and sit in my seat. What's the rush? We're headed to the farmers' market, for Pete's sake. The kale can wait another ten minutes.

I relax.

But Benji does not. And he does not budge. Let's face it, as strategies go, waiting out a two-year-old is just bananas.

I think of what good old Dr. Spock would say. I trust my son. Maybe he's trying to tell us something. He probably doesn't feel like being strapped in because his body needs to move, to get out some pent-up energy. Heck, if you tried to strap me to a chair, I'd resist, too. I'd run. So Benji and I walk a few blocks to get out some energy and stretch our bodies. Gwen drives alongside.

We have a lovely walk hand in hand. Benji is all smiles now, happy and delighted. A Norman Rockwell painting: Dad and son on Main Street.

A few blocks later Gwen pulls over. Surely Benji has moved on. We get in, and I try to buckle him into his car seat. But move on he has not. He is stiff as a board and crying. As if our Norman Rockwell moment never happened.

Just as I think we're going to have to go full-tilt Ferber on him, I remember to attune. To get mindful. To really pay attention. Benji's stuck. He's obsessed and lost in a tantrum. I ask myself, "What can help Benji relax and move on? What will interest him and fish him out of his mire?"

Answer: Well, he's been very social lately. He loves playing with friends.

So I ask him, "Benji, what's the name of your friend who's coming over later?"

On a dime, his body goes slack. He looks at me. We make eye contact.

"Greta," he says, catching his breath, focused on something new.

My face lights up. "Ohhhh, Greta," I say, as I buckle him into the car seat. He is smiling, happy as a clam.

Why did this work?

I have no idea. And no formula to repeat it.

Except to look closely at the moment. To be present and really pay attention. To respond not out of habit and not based on prior situations but directly to each new reality.

This, to me, is Conscious Parenting. But what does it entail? Should I bring the boys to kids' yoga? Use cloth diapers? No diapers? Cosleep? Keep a family bed? How many slings do I need to own?

What do we say when Benji throws his butternut squash against the wall? Or after Noah has a tough day at school? How do I avoid passing along my own anxieties and neuroses? And what the heck can Gwen and I do to stay connected amid the chaos?

Do we practice Attachment Parenting, Playful Parenting, Unconditional Parenting, or Simplicity Parenting? Or do I heed Lenore Skenazy's *Free-Range Kids* and back off and stop hovering, already!? Who knows, maybe sweet Dr. Spock got it right sixty years ago when he told us simply, "Trust yourself. You know more than you think you do."

Sometimes I think all I need to do is pose as a Republican for a decade or two so my kids will rebel and become hippie environmentalists.

To answer these pressing parenting questions, I have been reading books, watching countless videos, and attending workshops, seminars, and trainings. I have even worn a synthetic strap-on belly during downward dog posture.

In digging deep into all these approaches, I've found some solutions, yes, but equally important, as I've searched for the keys to Conscious Parenting, I've learned an awful lot about trust, compassion, and forgiveness — for myself and for my kids — and I think, in this, I may have stumbled on the very heart of yoga as well.

This process has involved an Ayurvedic doctor, a plus sign on a pregnancy test, an osteopathic shaman, the Eric Carle Museum, and not much sex. But before we get into all that, let's head over to the Kripalu Center for Yoga and Health in Lenox, Massachusetts, on a Friday in 2003, when I meet my wife and our tale begins.

Chapter 1

Before Babies

*P*arenting young children is not unlike serfdom.

Except that you're madly, wildly in love with your feudal lords.

As soon as the kids get a bit older you completely forget all this. You forget that for eight years you had given up eating sitting down and thinking clearly, and you start telling friends with younger children to "soak it in because it goes so fast."

These friends smile at you politely and probably know you're right, but secretly they want to grind their heel on your little toe. Just enough to cause you some pain but no serious damage.

By the time I wrote the last few chapters of this book, I too had forgotten all this. After reading that first draft, my editor, who has two young children, wanted to grind his heel on my toe. His comments contained words like *smug, facile*, and *throw this book against the wall*. Thankfully, he woke me up, and I revised the book. He reminded me that everyone except people with small children seems to know exactly how best to parent. It is much easier from the sidelines. But in the arena, it is just madness.

I had forgotten that when my boys were two and five, I felt ninety-seven years old. I remembered only the pure bliss of a bike ride together on a sunny, cloudless spring day. I forgot that for a few years, Gwen and I sat on different couches in the evening and mostly snapped at each other when we did speak.

It was not always like that, and it's not at all like that now between Gwen and me. It truly, as they say, gets better. Now we are on our honeymoon all over again.

But I'm getting ahead of myself.

I met Gwen — twice — at the Kripalu Center for Yoga and Health in the Berkshire Mountains of western Massachusetts. The first time I thought she was much too good for me, which she is, so I didn't pay much attention to her. A really excellent strategy, I know.

The second time, two years later, I was visiting my yoga teacher, as I did every four weeks. On September 5, 2003, I left Januar's office on the third floor, walked down the hallway, and peeked into Vairaigya.

Vairaigya was the small closet of a room in which Kripalu's long-term volunteers stashed leftovers from Saturday night's chocolate cake, surfed the Internet on an Apple IIe computer, and swapped clothes — residents could take or leave their Mexican serapes, quilted shirts from a Dead tour, and used Birkenstocks.

And sitting at the computer was Gwen.

I had not seen Gwen since I had moved out of Kripalu two years earlier. Back then we had interacted only a few times and had exchanged maybe ten words. We had different jobs at the ashram. I washed dishes in the kitchen and she worked in grounds and maintenance — shoveling walks, painting, and using power tools.

I had always had a crush on her but considered her simply out of my league: she was radiant and Canadian and had worked backcountry trail crew in Banff National Park.

But Gwen looked right at me and said, "Hi, *Brian*."

She knew my name! There was even a sparkle in her eye.

In my best Barry White, I replied, "Hey, Gwen. Wanna get some dinner together?"

To myself, though, I shrieked, "Holy shit, she knows my name. I think she likes me!"

We headed to the dining hall, flashed our name tags at the door greeter, gathered our trays of salad, pea soup, and mashed potatoes, and walked out to the patio overlooking the gorgeous Berkshire Mountains.

On any given night there are many more dinner dates happening at Kripalu than most people realize.

We sat together for hours until it was dark, and then we moved to an unoccupied yoga room — the typical second act for any Kripalu date. We talked there some more and then decided to walk in the dark to the lake.

We stopped at my car for a blanket and bumped into a mutual friend who still lived and worked at Kripalu. She eyed us and said, "Wow, two of my favorite people together. I didn't know you knew each other. Wait a minute. Are you in love?"

We blushed.

Before leaving to drive back to Northampton, I asked Gwen for her number. She wrote it down, smiled, planted a kiss on my cheek, and skipped back to the building. This is how Canadians are. Like in a continuous episode of *Anne of Green Gables*. To figure out the Canadian year, simply subtract fifty from the current year. Gwen was in 1953.

I don't believe in being coy or playing romantic games, so I called Gwen the next day. I invited her to dinner and a Ram Dass talk in Northampton. I'd make sushi before the talk.

Gwen showed up. And pretty much never left. We were inseparable. We hiked. We cooked organic meals. We did yoga and played strip Scrabble.

Gwen's contract at Banff National Park was over for the season, so in mid-October, she flew to Banff, packed up her car, and drove cross-country to move to Northampton.

I was a bit worried, though. Even under ideal circumstances, New England, or anywhere else in the world, would have a difficult time competing with Banff National Park's beauty and splendor. And I wanted Gwen to like Northampton. But late October, early November, is a particularly gray time in western Massachusetts. I'd have been far more confident of my chances in summer or during the white wonderland of January.

Despite the bare trees and gray-brown grass, Gwen stayed.

Later that month we traveled together to my friend Zach's wedding in Scottsdale, Arizona. I was going to propose during my best man toast, but Gwen just didn't seem ready. I know this because in our rental car en route from the airport to the tux shop, in casual conversation, Gwen said, "I'm just not ready." I stashed the diamond necklace in my coat pocket for the remaining six days of vacation.

One month later Gwen was ready, and on Christmas morning we got engaged. I had always wondered how I could one day have a wedding that would reflect my eclectic spiritual beliefs but not alienate my Jewish relatives from New Jersey. I needed a druid, a rabbi, and a swami to co-officiate. We settled for our environmentally conscious half-Jewish yoga teacher.

In fact, my family's expectations of me had changed after ten years of my nomadic yogic life spent ashram hopping, town hopping, and couch hopping. Now I think they were simply happy that I was getting married at all.

Plus, they were pleased that I wanted a fairly big wedding. Years earlier, my first Kripalu yoga teacher had given me some advice. Yolanthe had been married at sunset on a mountaintop in California in the 1970s. The ceremony was witnessed by only a few friends. They wore flower garlands and hippie dresses and were holding hands in a circle around the happy couple. (There were likely drugs involved.) Yolanthe and her husband divorced a few years later, and she had always wondered if a bigger, more involved wedding might have given them a better chance at staying married. Would more planning and ritual and support from friends and extended family have given them a more definitive start, a more grounded beginning? Would it have made them accountable to more people? Did they miss out on Great-Aunt Gertrude's scolding, "Divorce? But you just got married. And I flew in from Florida for the wedding. Out of the question."

I always remembered Yolanthe's advice. "Brian," she said in her Dutch accent that made everything sound like a military command, "Hev a beeg vedding! It gijh you a virm shtarting poynt. It shements your vouuuws!"

I could see what she meant. At my brother's wedding in 1994, I got to know my sister-in-law's family. I worked with her dad to transport the ketubah. We negotiated family photos for two very hungry hours. Decorating Larry and Pam's car, I bonded with their college friends. The wedding built community and lent gravity to Larry and Pam's vows.

Gwen and I were married under a giant oak tree. We wrote our own vows. We asked our community to participate. Our mothers lit a unity candle to symbolize the coming together of our families. Gwen's brother played keyboard, and her sister played cello. My friend Zach was emcee.

The reception was a blast. Though my gentile friends, in hoisting me up on a chair for the hora dance, seemed to misunderstand the tradition. They believed that their task was to buck me off — more Texas than Jewish. I held on for dear life. In the photos you can see the veins in my forehead as I clasp the chair. I think I left nail marks.

During the hora, things really heated up. The cooks from the local Blue Goose Café were preparing the feast and had a grease fire in the kitchen, which set off the fire alarm. My great aunt Litza was the first to hear it above the blaring "Hava Nagila."

Among more than one hundred family, friends, and guests dancing feverishly in concentric circles to *"Uru ahim belev-sameachhh,"* in a voice as loud as her seventy-five-year-old lungs could muster, Litza began shouting, "This place is on *fire!*"

My aunt Sandy, straining to hear her, replied, "Yeah, I know. It's *hopping!*"

"No," Litza insisted. "It's really *on fire!*"

Sandy should have understood Litza's meaning immediately. Seventy-five-year-old Jewish ladies in floral print dresses do not speak like Venus Flytrap from *WKRP in Cincinnati*.

The folks from the Blue Goose doused the fire and moved their operations to barbecues outside. We feasted on local free-range chicken and organic heirloom tomatoes. For dessert we ate wedding cake made from spelt flour and Sucanat instead of white sugar.

Gwen and I decided to travel around the country for our honeymoon, and we budgeted for three weeks. All this was a terrible mistake. We spent most of our time getting out west, and by the time we made it, we had to turn around for home. Things start to look a little different once you pass the Great Lakes. Until then, you might as well have taken a joyride back and forth twenty-three times across northern New Jersey.

When we got home I made a collage of mementos for Gwen. It still hangs somewhere in the bowels of the basement.

Chapter 2

Not Not Trying

*A*fter the honeymoon, I was reading Bill Bryson's *A Walk in the Woods*. I went to an outdoor store and bought a nice North Face ergonomic backpack and a light water bottle, and I started walking everywhere. I could take the hour and a half to walk somewhere that would take ten minutes in a car because I had the time.

One day I needed to take a check to the local newspaper for an advertisement, so I walked it over. I was exhilarated from the exercise, the fresh air, and my contribution to saving the planet. When I arrived, I sat in a chair beside the classified ad rep's cubicle to sign a paper and hand her the check. I was so excited to be there and to be alive and free.

I looked at her and said, "I just walked here from Florence!"

Silence.

"That's, like, four miles!"

Silence. She handed me a pen to sign my paperwork, eager to move on to the next sheet in her towering pile. Definitely a parent.

I, on the other hand, had unlimited time. Which was about to change.

Gwen and I had been married for six months, and we went for a routine visit to my Ayurvedic teacher in Boston. I was going to get a checkup and the potions for my yearly cleanse. It was difficult to leave this guy's office without a crate of decoctions, tinctures, and powders. But they worked. After every yearly cleanse, I felt more alert, creative, and vibrant than ever.

Gwen came along. I'd been seeing Farrukh for six years and we had become friends, and I wanted Gwen to meet him. Plus, she was interested in trying a cleanse.

I had my session first. He felt my Ayurvedic pulses. He looked at my tongue and my eyes. He asked me questions about my diet, the size of my bowel movements, and my sleep habits. And he prescribed a cleanse. I would drink three shakes a day and take a cocktail of herbal supplements to cleanse my liver and colon. I would eat from a prescribed diet of organic, simple, unprocessed foods. I'd avoid sugar and common food allergens such as wheat, dairy, and eggs. To give my body a break from its usual foods, he recommended a wide variety of low-mercury fish and prescribed rabbit and duck rather than chicken. I was excited. I knew I'd feel charged with energy.

Then it was Gwen's turn. She had been sitting next to me during my session, so we simply switched chairs. He took her pulses. He looked at her tongue and eyes. He asked her questions about her diet and sleep habits. I got to hear about her bowel movements.

Farrukh began tailoring a cleanse for Gwen, when, in passing, I mentioned that we might begin "trying" in a year or so. Farrukh stopped dead in his tracks. He went white and sweaty. As though visited from beyond, as though channeling, he told us that Gwen might not be able to get pregnant, and if she did, we would lose the fetus in the first trimester. He wanted her to have several hormone tests.

We stared ahead, pale and terrified, our stomachs in our shoes.

After the tests, which would cost four hundred dollars, we'd know more.

Gwen left with no cleanse.

We drove home in silence.

Finally, Gwen spoke. Her words woke us from our terror. "Wait a minute. What's he talking about? We don't know if there's really any problem."

"Right. What if he's wrong?" We were regaining our footing, soothing ourselves. We reached out for our previous reality, the one that did not include any terror of miscarriages and infertility.

"What if we just stop using birth control, and see what happens. We can do the hormone tests later if needed."

I agreed. We had not been planning on trying for another year anyway, so there was no rush. We decided to see what would happen before we dove into a cascade of interventions, even if the cascade consisted of holistic tests and natural treatments. After all, Gwen was in terrific health. She could climb mountains in a single Canadian bound. She could handle a chain saw and she ate brown rice and chard with eager gusto. Surely she was vibrantly healthy.

So we stopped not trying.

We went on official record with friends. If Facebook had existed back then, we'd have switched our birthing status from *not trying* to *not not trying*. We worried there might be some truth to Farrukh's fears and were not quite ready to commit to the actual designation of *trying*.

And back then, before we had kids, we didn't not try quite a bit. We didn't not try in the den. We'd not not try before a movie, during a movie, after the movie, in the kitchen, on the bed, under the bed. We not not tried with the zeal of newlyweds.

And all that not not trying paid off. Quickly. I actually know when we conceived. I had a feeling. And several days later Gwen was sure. She could feel the changes in her body. On a trip home to Northampton after visiting my parents in New Jersey, we stopped at a CVS and bought three pregnancy tests. One long pee later, we had three plus signs.

Chapter 3

A Squirrel in Our Bed

We were still worried about Farrukh's predictions, so we waited to tell friends and family. But when we confided in our one friend who was already a mom, she said, "Why wait? Tell people that you'd want to know if you were to lose the baby. You'd need their love and support. Why be isolated and alone?"

She was right, so we shared the news. And we waited together.

The first trimester passed. Gwen was healthy.

She was nauseous in the mornings. But she found that she just needed to stay well fed. If she ate small snacks all day, she was fine. I'd wake up at three in the morning in a start, thinking, "What's that noise?" Just as I was jumping up to fetch a broom to shoo the squirrel from our bed, I'd realize, "Oh, that's just Gwen propped up on three pillows and munching saltines in the dark."

A few weeks into the second trimester, we were confident enough to tour midwives in the area. Actually, first we toured the hospital. It was very nice and even had rooms with tubs for water births, but it was cold and sterile and we really wanted our baby to be born at home.

If you contemplate a home birth, everyone you know, from your mother to your mechanic, will ask, "But isn't home birth unsafe and totally insane?"

I don't think it is. In fact, if we look historically, home birth has been practiced in 99.999 percent of the births since humans began walking upright. Jimmy Carter was actually the first US president *not* to be born at home.

But what about safety?

In the UK, the very reputable National Institute for Health and Clinical Excellence reports that mortality during home births is the same as it is for hospital births. And Holland reports that a home birth led by a midwife "does not increase the risks of mortality among low-risk women." These Dutch know what they are talking about; in Holland, 30 percent of births occur at home.

The same report goes on to state that there is equality between home birth and hospital birth "provided the maternity care system facilitates this choice through the availability of well-trained midwives and through a good transportation and referral system." Translation: Home birth is great, as long as midwives are skilled and it's easy to get into the hospital when needed.

Maybe that's where the United States falls short. How can we have "well-trained midwives and a good transportation and referral system" to support home birth when the official stance of the American College of Obstetricians and Gynecologists is that "planned home birth is associated with a twofold to threefold increased risk of neonatal death when compared with planned hospital birth"?

I'm no conspiracy theorist, but in a capitalistically driven health-care system, how can doctors and hospitals possibly support home birth? Profits are made in the hospital, not in homes. Interestingly, the acronym for the American College of Obstetricians and Gynecologists is A-COG. I'm just saying.

Thankfully, where Gwen and I live is an exception. Northampton is an enclave of holistic hippie culture. A time capsule to 1850. You can see why a Canadian would be comfortable here. I half expect to see Pa rolling the pony trap into town every morning. So we have excellent home-birth midwives and hospital support systems in case of emergency.

By the way, whereas the American College of Obstetricians and Gynecologists is A-COG, the United Kingdom's National Institute for Health and Clinical Excellence is, appropriately, NICE. To which I concur. The fine chaps at NICE report that women who give birth at home are

1. more likely to deliver vaginally.
2. more likely to have greater satisfaction from their birth experience than women who gave birth in a hospital.
3. more likely to avoid hospital interventions such as analgesia and a delivery using instruments.

Other countries certainly have a thing or two to teach us in this arena. In Australia, health insurance covers home birth. In Canada, the Ministry of Health actually recommends home births. And the UK's parliamentary undersecretary for health, Lord Hunt himself, has sired two babies born at home.

The very founder of obstetrics in the United States, Joseph DeLee, the man who considered birth a medical crisis to be carried out only in hospital, recanted by the end of his life, warning mothers, "Mother Nature's methods of bringing babies are still the best."

When I went for my weekly visit to Donna, my psychotherapist, she was appalled at our home-birth decision. Terrified for me, she said, "But hospital midwives have seen thousands of births. They simply know more. You're putting your baby in jeopardy."

This rattled me. I was resolute but, apparently, not totally confident. So I took a break from my sessions with Donna.

Gwen and I interviewed home-birth midwives. The first midwife we met was lovely, perfect, really, but she lived forty-five minutes away, so we passed.

The next midwife was also lovely, but her house, where we met, was shockingly filthy. Dirty socks and dirty dishes and dirt, and it smelled. I'm not a slave to the OCD sterilize-everything dragon of mainstream hospitals, but come on. Her name, by the way, was Ruth Ann Uterise. Not sure if that was her original name. If so, I guess she was truly born for this job.

Looking back, I see now that Ruth Ann's house was not really so filthy. It's just that she had kids. These days, it's not unusual at all in my house to see a pair of undies on the kitchen counter or an apple slice decaying under a bed. And on a warm day, you could encounter all number of smells wafting about the house. I probably owe Ruth Ann an apology.

The third midwife, Wendy, seemed perfect. Her office was close by, she was confident and incredibly experienced, and she had a tidy office. We signed on.

And I must say that sessions with Wendy were everything healthcare should be. She listened intently. She trusted Gwen and her body's messages. Gwen felt heard and empowered. And Wendy knew her stuff. She was noninvasive. Rather than a Doppler, she used a fetoscope (basically a very powerful stethoscope) to listen to the baby's heart, and she could tell where the baby was by intuition and palpation, with just a feel of Gwen's belly. Most mainstream doctors have lost this skill.

Wendy was absolutely perfect...for Gwen. But I soon realized that while she deeply respected women, maybe she resented men and husbands just a bit. And, really, with good reason, since men have basically stolen her vocation and made it all but illegal to practice her art at home. I did not quite see it that first day, but I had entered the den of the Amazons. I should have picked up on this when everyone else in the room (all women) was led to a cushy chair, leaving only a small, wooden footstool for me. I had to crane my neck to see what was happening. I might as well have been dressed in an oversize onesie and diapered.

After a few sessions I noticed this happening, but I was so in awe of Gwen and her growing belly that I just considered my time in the sessions as prostrating at the feet (literally) of the goddess.

Gwen's belly grew.

And grew.

And grew.

We followed the size and look of the fetus in two different parenting books. We followed it through its raisin size and watched the pictures as it became a plum. Gwen commented that the book must have been written by a pregnant woman, because all the descriptions were of foods. We read the books and visualized our olive-sized baby's tiny fingers developing, amazingly at only six or seven weeks!

We bought our own fetoscope to listen to our baby's heart. These things are like torture devices. The ear buds are so hard. My ears hurt even now just thinking about them. It cost $98 and made me feel like a real home-birther. But I never once found the heartbeat. Our midwife could look at Gwen's belly and somehow divine exactly where and at what angle to place the chest piece, but I never once found the sweet spot. We passed the fetoscope along to friends. They returned it to us, reporting the same results.

So what about Farrukh? What of his stark warnings? I'm not sure, but I've experienced this sort of thing several times. My eye doctor told me just last month that my new glasses could unhinge my sight, and if so, I'd need weekly eye treatments. She just forgot to say that there was a 0.0001% chance of that happening. And natural practitioners and esoteric folks are even worse. A psychic friend once told me that my next relationship would be with a man. She was wrong. An aura reader once predicted that I'd have a very bad experience with a Dachshund. So far incorrect.

This, of course, is not to dis natural health practitioners or even psychics. It's just that they can sometimes be wrong. Or maybe, as in the movie *The Matrix*, they tell us exactly what we need to hear at that very moment. Maybe, for example, Noah was ready to be born and spoke through Farrukh to get those pesky latex condoms out of his way.

Chapter 4

Birthing Class

*G*wen and I attended a parent education class. It was held at a
holistic health clinic in the area. One of the clinic's special-
ties was chelation therapy. Chelation is a controversial treatment
in which a patient with heavy metal toxicity sits in a chair for four
hours while chelating agents drip into his or her blood to remove the
toxins.

This therapy is used in mainstream medicine in cases of heavy-
metal poisoning. It is used by alternative medical providers as a
treatment for autism and heart disease. This clinic specializes in the
alternative uses — I don't think the small town of Northampton,
Massachusetts, would require twelve dedicated chelation stations
for folks who've gone and swallowed their thermometer or recently
handled plutonium. Each "station" is actually a La-Z-Boy recliner
outfitted with an IV drip, a magazine rack, and a remote to the near-
est TV set.

The chelation room was the only space in the facility large
enough for our meetings. So we'd meet there and sit in the recliners

and rest our arms on the IV drips. It was a bit austere and medical for about-to-pop home-birthing moms and dads.

The woman who ran the session was bubbly and jolly, and the class was informative, but ultimately, of course, it failed to prepare us for labor and parenting. Which isn't at all the teacher's fault. You see, until we have children of our own, we are incapable of understanding what birth and parenting are really like. If you are not yet a parent, and you are reading this, your mind censors it. It's like a covenant with God. All you see is something like, "Yum, aren't kids *sooo* cute!"

In fact, a colleague with two small children responded flatly to our happy news with, "Life as you know it is over." We didn't believe him. We just thought, "Poor jaded fellow."

Our teacher even showed us videos of labor and birthing, but we just nodded blithely, imagining that complications only happen to other people. People who don't do yoga or eat multiple daily servings of quinoa.

I retain two vivid memories of class. The first is that, man, those pregnant ladies can eat. Like wolves. There'd be sushi and melon and kale chips and chicken legs and chocolate pudding passed around as we watched birthing footage and practiced breathing.

The other thing I remember is that the teacher told us that if we don't circumcise our baby boy and one day he asks us, "Why am I different from dad?" we can just say, "We didn't want to hurt you."

Gwen's blood work showed that she was anemic. The midwives wouldn't do a home birth unless her iron count was at least 10.5. So we took aggressive steps to raise her iron.

Our plan: Blackstrap molasses in her morning cereal, shitake mushrooms at lunch, red meat and kale daily, nettles tea and medical-grade molasses cookies for dessert, and daily natural iron supplements, especially Floradix.

After several months, she was retested and we squeaked by at 10.7.

When Gwen was six months pregnant we moved from our apartment to a house. I read in a feng shui book that as a baby grows in its mama's belly, its spirit gathers below the mother's bed. On moving day, I got down under the bed with a baking tin and told our baby, whom at this point we called Sweetie Pie, to hop in. In case he or she was asleep, I swept in all the dust bunnies. I explained that we were moving and left the new address, along with a map, under the bed for any stragglers. Most of our stuff went into the truck, but I carried Sweetie Pie on my lap in the car.

Gwen was getting close, and at this point we received many, many pieces of advice. And lots of opinions regarding home birth and birthing in general. The most important being:

When friends want to share their birth story with you, especially when they begin with, "Well that's nothing, I was..." feel free to slam on the brakes. If you have attended five births and relish this sort of story, fine. Otherwise, show them the palm of your outstretched hand and stop them midsentence. Just explain, "I don't want to alarm myself."

That said, I'm about to tell you all about Gwen's six-day labor. Of course, this is a special situation that would never happen to you. But, if you're feeling sensitive, please skip to page 29.

Chapter 5

Six Days of Labor

*D*ay 1: In the middle of watching a DVD of *Meet the Fockers*, Gwen has a contraction. I grab a pencil and the closest thing to write on (oddly, a scrap of wood) and begin timing.

Five minutes apart and lasting one minute! Wahoo! Make the call!

We call Wendy.

I unlock the front door and gather our birthing paraphernalia.

I unfold the nylon birthing tub on the carpet in the family room and prepare to fill it.

Wendy, her assistant midwife, and their apprentice arrive.

They take one look at Gwen...and...no sale.

"Go back to bed. Let things percolate some more."

Day 2: Pretty much the same thing, except that this time we are reading *The Hobbit* to each other when contractions peak. Bilbo has just been captured by the trolls.

I suggest that Gwen try sounding during contractions. In yoga lingo, *sounding* means making noise, often moaning, to release tension and allow emotion and energy to flow. I had heard once that making sounds can lessen the intensity of pain.

Gwen starts moaning. But I think maybe the noise is causing her more stress than relaxation. I know it surely is for me. Our house sounds like a war hospital. I sit powerlessly for hours listening to Gwen suffer.

Day 3: Gwen is laboring but not progressing. Her contractions are sometimes very strong as in active labor and sometimes much weaker. Gwen and I march up and down the stairs to stimulate labor. We go for a hike in the woods. We sway and moan together to a Krishna Das CD.

The midwives give Gwen a homeopathic remedy to move things along. It does not work. They don't realize that Canadians who have lived in the woods and used power tools are immune to anything as subtle as homeopathic medicine.

Day 4: Gwen is sounding and we are not sleeping. I sneak into the basement to call my sister to cry, get support, and find a moment of normalcy.

Today the midwives give Gwen herbal tinctures. And they finally give me a role. I am sent out to buy castor oil. The same quality that makes castor oil open the poop chute can bring about the peristalsis of labor.

When castor oil fails, I am given a second role. Male semen contains prostaglandins, a hormonelike secretion that happens to help the cervix dilate. Plus an orgasm in a pregnant mama releases oxytocin, which, if the body is ready, can bring about or strengthen contractions.

We are sent into the bedroom with assurances that the midwives will be out of earshot. Honestly, by this point, we have lost all sense of modesty and are so wearied that we would think nothing of having sex right in front of the midwives. We'd have coupled on Fox News without a second's thought. Our only thought is to meet our baby.

We retire to the bedroom. But we are exhausted and scared. Have you ever tried to have loving, sensual sex when exhausted and terrified?

My mind is churning and I am barely present in my body. And to be fair, Gwen is in no mood, either. I do the best I can. But come on, even on a good day, I have to focus to hit the fifteen-minute mark.

I do not earn an A on this assignment. We emerge three minutes later with heads hung low. No orgasm and no labor.

Day 5: Gwen is still laboring but not progressing. Morale sinks and we lose hope. We are bathed in exhaustion and fear. I attempt to stifle my fears that Gwen is dying.

An acupuncturist pays us a house call. Gwen lies on our bed and the acupuncturist sticks her with needles. She fills one with herbs and lights it on fire. This is called moxibustion. The acupuncturist leads us in song and chant. She exudes TLC and brings sweetness and love back into the house.

By the time the acupuncturist leaves, Gwen and I are renewed. We march the stairs once more, now with the acupuncturist's mantra, "I am a hollow bamboo, open up and let the babe flow through." We repeat this a thousand times, and we push on for yet another day.

At this point, I realize that our midwives would eat me if this sort of thing were legal and socially acceptable. At best, they see me as a nuisance, as a doofy pre–*Modern Family* Phil Dunphy. At worst, they seem to feel that I am feeding Gwen hostile intel. Disempowering her. Telling her she can't do it. They tell me I need to work on my anger problem.

I'm pretty sure I don't have an anger problem. And I know that I am not disempowering Gwen. Just the opposite — I am in awe of her. But the midwives are not really speaking to me; they are talking to the generations of men who had stolen their profession and put laboring women on their backs (a terrible birthing position, convenient only for the physician) to be drugged, told what to do, and hidden from their birthing baby by a sterile sheet in a hospital. I am not these men.

"What do husbands usually do during labor?" I ask.

"You know, they usually eat an egg salad sandwich and watch the game in the TV room." Gwen and I have no TV room. Only a yoga room with an altar. Though I do enjoy a nice egg salad sandwich on gluten-free bread.

Just like Gwen and me, the midwives are scared. The following day — day six — the team asks Gwen if she wants to go to the hospital. They do not want my input. If they would only ask, though, my input would be precisely, "Gwen, what do your body and the baby need?" Gwen takes a walk outside in the fresh snow to consider her options. It's a miracle, really, that she can still stand.

Gwen does not ultimately get to make her decision, though, because she comes back during her walk for a pee break and spots meconium in the amniotic fluid.

Meconium is the fancy name for baby poop. Ordinarily the fetus retains the meconium and releases it upon birth. Early release of meconium into the amniotic fluid indicates potential fetal distress (like pooping your pants when stressed). Fetal distress is alarming in and of itself. But even more important, you do not want the baby to inhale the poop into its lungs — babies in utero breathe amniotic fluid, not air.

The midwives tell me to pack clothes. They will drive us to the hospital. In home-birth lingo this is called transporting.

I break down and cry. I had so wanted our baby to be born at home.

I walk around weeping as I gather a few sacred objects for Gwen. A photo of her scaling Cascade Mountain in the Canadian Rockies. Mala beads. A candle.

As we wait in the car for the midwives to gather their tools and close up our house, Gwen, too, finally cries. She cries of exhaustion, of disappointment, and, actually, of relief to be moving forward.

Chapter 6

Thanksgiving

*W*e drive to the hospital on Thanksgiving Day, through an early winter blizzard. Wendy has a plan with the midwives at the hospital for cases such as this, but there is an error in the paperwork, so we must be admitted through the emergency room. I wait in line and fill out bureaucratic paperwork. Wendy warns me to keep my anger in check.

Wendy tells us that she can only give certain advice in the hospital and that she will have to defer to the staff.

We settle into a room. The hospital midwife examines Gwen. She can give us three hours to progress and then she'll need to intervene. Gwen marches. She chants. Wendy waves us into the bathroom for more sex.

We have moved from homeopathics, to herbs, to castor oil, to acupuncture. Inducing labor through pharmaceutical Pitocin is the next step.

The hospital midwife gives Gwen three successive doses of Pitocin to get her into active labor. I forgot to tell the doctors that Gwen is Canadian. One-fifth that dose would have gotten a neurotic

Jew from New Jersey into gear, but a Canadian of farmer blood needs much more.

The hospital midwife also reaches in and adjusts the baby's positioning, which helps free him or her up and allows labor to progress.

Gwen, as I've told you, is hearty. She's the one in an action movie who keeps running after taking five arrows in the leg. She's like Walter Payton running for a TD with five defenders on his back. She's like Gwen, and that's quite something. In fact, once labor advances, miraculously, Gwen finds the energy to push the baby out.

The midwife has a small basin of oil right on the hospital bed and massages Gwen's perineum throughout the pushing. This is a big baby with a nice-sized noggin, and that oil helps an awful lot both to get him out and to prevent Gwen from tearing. Using oil during labor is no different from using it to get a stuck ring off a finger. It's not rocket science. Oil helps. A lot.

You can even prep the perineum for the big stretch with gentle oil massage for months before the birth. What a solution! Simple. Elegant. Genius. Sometimes modern allopathic medicine is so clever. And sometimes so barbaric. A little oil and massage can prevent a lot of pain and several weeks of needing to sit on a pillow. Plus, think about it. You're getting ready for bed and out comes the oil for perineal massage. This can only end very, very well.

As soon as Noah is out, the midwife whisks him over to the pediatrician's station, set up a few feet away. Noah has to be examined for meconium in his lungs. I want him to connect with Gwen and me immediately, to know he is safe and loved and welcome in the world, so I coo to him the whole time, "Hello Sweetie Pie, I'm your dad, and that's mom, and we're so glad you've chosen us. We love you, little sweetie!"

The doctors aspirate Noah's nose and mouth and use a fiber-optic tube to make sure that his lungs are poop-free.

No meconium. He is perfectly healthy.

After the exam I cut the cord and when no one is looking I smear the blood on my jeans as a keepsake. The pediatrician catches this and shakes his head. I imagine he is thinking, "Dirty home-birthers."

The pediatrician hands Noah to me and I carry our little baby to Gwen for his first nurse. Gwen is beaming.

We take home Noah's placenta. The nurses wrap it for us in blue hospital paper. They don't even ask; they know that home-birthers who transport to the hospital bring home the placenta.

We store it at the bottom of our freezer. This leaves me concerned that a visiting friend will find it and surprise us with dinner. Really, I'm shocked that the *Meet the Fockers* film franchise has not mined this scenario. They've already milked foreskin, breasts, and Robert De Niro's erect penis. I'd think eating placenta would be the logical next gag.

A few months later, we have a lovely ceremony and plant the placenta under an oak tree sapling. The tree looks great. Noah recently told a visitor, "See that tree. Know why it's so healthy? It's 'cause of my 'centa!"

The labor took a total of six days. Which is called stalled or prodromal labor and happens very rarely. I surely would have succumbed to nervous exhaustion on day two. I must say, and not for the last time, thank God, or Goddess, that Gwen is the female in our household — I never could have done it.

Chapter 7

The Phlebotomist

*A*s soon as Noah is born, I am all love. I am surrounded and enveloped by it. There is no other feeling. I appreciate everyone in the room — even the hospital's pediatrician, who had been loudly discussing the Red Sox's pitching staff with the phlebotomist as they waited in the wings for Gwen to push Noah out.

I'm glad we started at home. And I'm very thankful for the nurse midwife at the hospital who got him out.

We live for a few days like a king, queen, and baby prince. Friends and family from all over come to meet and kiss baby Noah. They bring gifts and food. Our friends Jeff and Amy bring knishes from New Jersey. My folks bring the best pizza I have ever tasted.

We opt to have Noah sleep in the room with us rather than in the nursery. And we don't use the bassinette the hospital offered. Noah sleeps right in the cot with Gwen. This makes her sleep lightly, feeling for him or waking to watch him breathe, but she doesn't mind. She is alight with love.

The next morning, the phlebotomist comes in. This is a tough occupation. Worse than being a dentist or even a parking ticket lady.

Phlebotomists have one and only one job. They jab people with needles. That may not sound too bad if you think of the one shot you got three years ago. But what if you gave that shot every day, all day. What if you had to make babies cry, children cringe, and adults sweat all day every day. This is a job with which Göring or Eichmann would have been thrilled.

So when Noah is but a few hours old, Göring comes in to do the heel prick. He places Noah naked on a cold metal scale and, of course, Noah cries. The phlebotomist pricks, and no blood. He pricks again. He pricks a third time. No blood. He massages Noah's leg and, no lie, turns him upside down. Finally blood. He smears it onto the Guthrie card, licks his lips, and heads out to his next victim. I'm convinced there will be lasting psychological scarring.

In the hospital, a nurse comes in every two hours to weigh Noah and record his nursings, pees, and poops. Does this make sense to you? Is nature this ignorant that it is unsafe to let mom and baby sleep and nurse on their own schedule for a night? Later we discover that we could have opted out of night check-ins. I had no idea. This is like suddenly learning that you could simply have asked for more allowance as a child.

We are trapped at the hospital for three days. The doctor is concerned about Noah's bilirubin levels, so we are under hospital lockdown. We try to contact our primary-care doc to sign us out under his watch, but it is Thanksgiving weekend, so he is unavailable and there is only one doctor on call for the whole county.

There never was a problem, but it's amazing to live in the space of feeling like there is. You can forget that there is only the possibility of a problem, not an actual problem. By day three, I was, of course, shouting conspiracy theory and raving mad. Maybe Wendy was right about my anger problem.

After three days we head home. I don't want Noah to be surprised by the transition, so I talk him through the whole affair.

Literally. It's like a mindfulness meditation or a Dick and Jane novel as I narrate our every step. "Noah, sweetie, you are going home with Mama and Dada to your house. I am picking you up now. Say good-bye to our hospital room... We are going down in the elevator. We are leaving the hospital... This is your car seat. I'm buckling you in. Mama is sitting right next to you... We're driving home now."

We want to practice the Continuum Concept, in which baby stays in contact skin-to-skin with mom or dad from birth until crawling, but I just don't think the Ye'kuana Indians of South America had to deal with mandated car seats and a drive home from the hospital. Still, Gwen coos and strokes Noah the whole way. Like every other new parent, I drive home on the freeway at seventeen miles an hour.

In the end, I'm not sure that Wendy was so wrong about birthing being left to the women. Men and women might just have a very different skill set. Birthing is not a time for a let's-fix-it approach. It's not a time for the hunters. It requires complete surrender. Surrender in the mother to the forces of nature. Surrender in her to relax and allow her body to birth the baby. Surrender, sometimes, to pain. Surrender of plans and expectations. And, above all, surrender to reality as it unfolds in its unique way.

For those six days of laboring and three days in the hospital, I got to see Gwen in her true power. She accomplished a miracle and made life.

I think birthing may indeed be for women, but still, I'm very glad to have been there. It was magic. And it was transformational. A firm reminder of the power of the human body. A firm reminder of the power and mystery of nature. A firm reminder that there is peace in surrender.

Chapter 8

Sweet Baby Lemongelo

Today you are You, that is truer than true.
There is no one alive who is Youer than You.

— Dr. Seuss, *Happy Birthday to You!*

*P*iece of advice. Don't tell anyone the name of your baby until your baby is born. Not even your cousin, who is like a best friend. Because before your baby is born, people will have no qualms about sharing their opinions with you. They will tell you any number of nasty stories about serial killers, psychos, and literary villains of the same name.

But once your baby is born and is sitting there squeaking and moving around like a baby dinosaur from *Jurassic Park*, people will say, "Ohh, hedo 'ittle sweet baby *Lemongelo*. What a sweet name. I just want to eat you up. Aren't you perfect!"

Okay, Lemongelo was a bad example. But you get the point.

My mom and dad each wanted us to name the baby after someone on their side of the family, a wish I wanted to accommodate. I think there is tremendous power in ancestors. I believe that they watch over us, help us, and invest us with power. But I needed Kissinger to negotiate the operation. What if we had only one child? Would we name after my side or Gwen's? If my side, then my mom's or my dad's?

In our family, Gwen is the researcher. She read all 476 pages of *The New American Dictionary of Baby Names* — cover to cover, like Rain Man reading the phone book. In considering each name, she developed a complex algorithm involving etymology, sound, current popularity, projected future popularity, potential nicknames, and suitability in Canada. The name George Bush, for example, does not go over well there.

So she'd comb the baby-name books and come to me with a list. Then I'd eliminate a few and we'd discuss the rest. If Noah had been a girl, he'd have been Hannah. For a while he was going to be Samuel, but then one of our closest friends had a baby and scooped the name. We chose Noah because we both liked its strong biblical power. Plus, when I was bar mitzvahed in New Jersey in 1984, the Noah story was my Torah portion. On my side, the *H* at the end honored my paternal grandpa, Herman, and we went with Samuel as the middle name, so *S* for my maternal grandma, Sylvia.

Choosing a name is important. But even if you screw up horrendously, kids can recover. Look at celebrity yogi Rod Stryker. Here's a powerful, charismatic, very successful yoga teacher. He was married to supermodel Cheryl Tiegs. He wrote a bestselling book. A truly inspiring man, with self-confidence and a beautiful heart. But at birth he was named Nimrod Gross. What were his parents thinking? Maybe they didn't speak English, and Nimrod is a beautiful name in the old country with no Urkel-like connotations.

I do think, though, that Rod overcompensated just a bit. His new name could costar with Buck Naked for all sorts of lascivious adult adventures. It sounds like what Ike Turner should have called himself.

By the way, Rod is actually the close friend of a friend, and I'm just playing around here at his expense. Rod, you are truly a sweet and inspiring man and a fabulous yoga teacher, and I intend to ask you to endorse this book.

Like Rod Stryker, I, too, have a much-improved name. I consider myself very lucky to be called Brian Leaf. It's a fine name for an eco-friendly parenting memoirist. It rolls off the tongue, is easy to pronounce, is loved by radio DJs, and sounds like I'm part druid. This is yet another debt I owe to my father. You see, he came to this country in the 1940s as Manny Lifschutz. When his elementary school classmates pronounced his name phonetically, *Lifshuts*, my dad would correct them, "No, no, no, it's Lif-*shits*." And they'd laugh. He recently told me, "Even my teachers laughed." He learned that *shit* was not as melodious here as it is in mother Austria.

As soon as my dad was old enough, in an inspiring act of foresight, adaptability, and courage, he changed his name, and the Leaf dynasty was born.

So here again, and not for the last time, thanks, Dad. You are my hero.

Chapter 9

The Myth of Smegma

I coulda been a kosher butcher like my brother.
The money's good. There's a union, with benefits.
And cows have no families. You make a mistake with a cow,
you move on with your life.

— Shakey the moyle, *Seinfeld*, "The Bris"

'm a bit distracted right now. Concerned that someone sitting near me in the café can see that I've written *smegma* at the top of the page. I think I saw Noah's babysitter come in earlier. I'm going to look over my shoulder to see who's sitting behind me.

I'm also depressed. Wendy gave me a book about circumcision. I've started the book and can't put it down. I'm not sure that I'll ever fully recover.

The book tells me

1. that circumcision took away length and girth from my penis.
2. that I would enjoy sex more if I had a foreskin.

You do not say these things to a man. Ever. Especially anything about size. Men freak out when size is mentioned. It's why every porno contains the phrase "Oh, you're sooo big." It's an aphrodisiac.

I'm trying to climb out of the hole. I tell myself that most men in the United States are circumcised, so it's a level playing field. It just means that uncircumcised men are heroes and that we are at a disadvantage when we leave the country.

Which we are. Around 70 to 85 percent of men in the world right now are *not* circumcised. You might be thinking, 70 to 85 percent is a pretty wide spread; why don't we have a better gauge on this number? Good question. The answer: there are a lot of penises to count and, mostly, they are covered up.

Besides size, the book brings up the issue of sex. Would I enjoy sex more if I had a foreskin?

I don't know. I like sex. I think it's pretty great. Really great. I wish I was having sex right now. But apparently I'd enjoy it a whole lot more if I still had my foreskin. The book tells me that the foreskin is like an eyelid protecting the sensitive mucous membrane of the upper shaft and head of the penis. Circumcision removes this protective skin, so that the skin underneath keratinizes, meaning it hardens and desensitizes, like a callus.

This much is science. But keep in mind that the rest is theory. Whether or not sex is less pleasurable without a foreskin is, of course, very difficult to test. How can Tobias from college who still has his foreskin (lucky dog!) tell me how sex feels different for him than it does for me?

I suppose the only one who really knows is Abraham himself, circumcised with a blunt stone at age ninety-nine. But he's not talking.

And nobody is lining up for a double-blind controlled study: Have sex. Rate it on a scale from 1 to 10. Then lose the foreskin, heal, have sex again with the same partner, and rate it again from 1 to 10. Any takers?

So it's difficult to test the reduced-pleasure hypothesis. And people don't talk about it much, so we don't gather much anecdotal evidence, either. Unless you are a professional sex worker or my friend Adeline, you probably rarely talk about sex, especially the specifics. I don't even know which of my friends have a foreskin and which don't. Maybe I'll ask the question on Facebook: "Share or Like if you have a foreskin."

Lately it's all I can think about. Yesterday I was headed to lunch, walking down Main Street in town, and I saw a baby boy and wondered, "So, kid, do you still have it?" I hope he does.

Worse than books are chat rooms. DO NOT VISIT CIRCUMCISION CHAT ROOMS. Seriously. These folks are pissed off. And quite deviant. One guy wraps bologna around his wiener to simulate a foreskin.

One man mentioned that he didn't know he was missing it until a girlfriend showed him the scar on his penis. To tell you the truth, neither did I, until I read Wendy's book. I knew about circumcision but never pondered the specifics or why I have a ring of discolored tissue around the shaft of my penis.

I am not dissing Abraham or my heritage. I suspect that three thousand years ago making a covenant to give a piece of our flesh to God made sense. That was a very different time. A time in which people hunted, and ate ox heart. But now, at the dawning of the Age of Aquarius, things, I think, are different. A subtler sacrifice would work just fine. An email, maybe. A text with a photo. Who knows, a tweet. It might be enough simply to light a candle and offer an appreciation.

According to yoga philosophy, the past age, the ascending Kali Yuga, was characterized, basically, by hitting each other with clubs. We can expect a bit more from the next stage, the Dvapara Yuga. In this stage, hopefully, we can stop cutting each other's penises as if it were a frat prank. What do you think old Abraham would say if he realized that he missed out by only a few thousand years? "D'oh!"

We all know about circumcision's Jewish roots in the covenant between God and Abraham, but whom do we have to thank for the mass popularization of circumcision? When did it cross the gentile line? In Victorian England, of course. Yes, the same folks who made sex and farting socially unacceptable. Will Ferrell and Judd Apatow owe Queen Victoria big-time. What if nudity, masturbation, and farting weren't funny?

In the 1800s, germ theory was gaining attention and people believed circumcision could fight the ultimate germ demon, *smegma*. Sounds like a Batman villain. They incorrectly believed smegma to be a breeding ground of bacteria. Somehow this theory persisted into modern-day New Jersey because I distinctly remember my middle school health teacher putting the fear of God into us. I recall sitting through a very uncomfortable lecture about uncircumcised boys folding back their foreskin to clean the white stuff with a Q-tip. This is hogwash, like telling someone to pull back their eyelid to wipe the eyeball. I'd have hated to be one of the few uncircumcised fellows in the group. We looked around the room, thinking, "Barbarians!"

Smegma is actually found in most animal genitalia and serves, in fact, to clean and lubricate the genitals, moistening the sensitive mucous membrane between the foreskin and the penis. The word *smegma* itself is Greek for *soap*.

Where the hell was Freud for all this? What would he have said about these wealthy white doctors all happily enjoying their foreskins while recommending that new babies lose theirs?

Circumcision was the new snake oil. It was touted to prevent or cure syphilis, epilepsy, hernia, headache, clubfoot, alcoholism, gout, and, god forbid, masturbation! This last one is not rocket science. He's been masturbating. Let's make his penis totally raw and see if he keeps it up. As I read older parenting books, I am absolutely astonished at how often people bring up masturbation. They were obsessed! "We must stop this epidemic!" I suppose things have changed. Just last night I watched Seth Rogen masturbate right on screen at the cinema.

Wendy's book posits that angry nuns promoted circumcision as punishment for masturbating tweens. This image disturbed me more than any other in the book. So I will share it with you. Sorta like, "Oy vey, this spoiled yoghurt is terrible! Here, try it…" So picture this. A sad, lonely orphan is caught masturbating. He is circumcised. And now he sits, huddled in a corner, quietly sobbing and holding his sore penis. Can you visualize that? Now I'm sobbing.

Another part of the book posits that we Jews kept up the practice so that men would remain faithful to their wives, since, *obviously*, sex with a circumcised penis is not that appealing anyway. Save me!

Okay, so if you have a penis and you are missing your foreskin, what to do? Well, according to the book, many such men opt for foreskin restoration surgery. Do they graft skin from the sensitive knee pit? No. From the scrotum. Of course. The other option is to stretch the remains of the foreskin at the circumcision scar. Over time it actually lengthens.

By the way, you owe me one for researching this stuff. Can you imagine the spam I'm going to get now that I've Googled "foreskin restoration"? Google analytics has likely placed me in a whole new unsavory category.

Lots of folks defer the decision of whether or not to circumcise to the thinking of the American Academy of Pediatrics. Seems sensible. But this organization is about as scientifically sound on this matter as Steve Martin's Theodoric of York, Medieval Barber. The AAP has flip-flopped on the matter at least four times. In 1971 the academy officially concluded that it was not a medical necessity. In 1989 they announced that there were good medical reasons for it. In 1999 they were neutral, stating in a report that the health benefits of the procedure were slim. And most recently, in 2012, the AAP changed their official stance, saying that the health benefits of circumcision outweigh the risks.

One of the founders of the American Medical Association, Lewis Sayre, in the late 1800s started recommending circumcision to cure paralysis and gross motor problems. He believed that a tight foreskin threw off the nervous system. "Hmm, this patient is paralyzed. Must be a tight penis."

All this is another perfect example of why we must, in parenting as in life, gather data, but ultimately stay grounded and follow our own hearts and intuition.

The livid anticircumcision set cites many reasons for their stance.

One is that circumcision creates the risk of meatal stenosis, a condition in which scar tissue blocks the urethra opening, making urination painful. I have a friend who remembers a traumatic operation when he was six in which the doctor had to cut his urethra opening because it was too small. Trying to get him to relax, the doctor said, "This won't hurt a bit," and then sliced.

Apparently, circumcisions have a median complication rate of 1.5 percent for newborns, with the most common complications being bleeding, infection, and the removal of either too much or too little foreskin. Circumcision advocates proudly report that "significant acute complications are rare," occurring in about one in five hundred procedures in the United States. That doesn't sound so rare to me. How long does it take five hundred babies to be born in the United States? One hour. So wait for it, wait for it…now. We just had a significant acute circumcision complication. And while we were waiting we had seven minor complications.

In the end, as you may have guessed, Gwen and I chose not to circumcise. People ask me, "What will you tell your son when he asks why his penis is different from yours?" I don't understand this concern. Why must his penis match mine? Our hair color is different. We have different noses (his distinctly Canadian, mine Jewish). His teeth are better than mine. Should he get braces and a retainer to mimic my overbite?

And what of my family? I grew up not religious but still very

Jewish. We ate bagels and lox, my grandma would bring over chicken soup when I was sick, and I like a latke as much as, maybe more than, the next guy. But my parents never asked if we were circumcising. By now they knew not to ask questions whose answers might be disappointing. And, frankly, I think they were just happy that I stopped following the Grateful Dead, that I married, and that we have a baby.

Ironically, for me, the decision actually did come down to God. I trust her, and I don't think she designed the human body with a throwaway foreskin, like an Old Navy tag we're supposed to remove before wearing. I think the human body is holy and magical and perfect as is.

Chapter 10

The Womanly Art of Breastfeeding

I get a kick out of that title, *The Womanly Art of Breastfeeding*. This is the name of the book published by La Leche League, and it's the bible of breastfeeding. The maxim for mammilla. The tome for teats.

What can I say? The title of the book makes me giggle.

Whenever I tell Gwen that the title amuses me, she looks at me as if I've just called Canada the fifty-first state or let out a very large, wet belch.

I just think there's something funny and awkward about the title. Not about breastfeeding. Breastfeeding is the bomb. It's dope.

There seem to be multiple camps to many things. There are Democrats and Republicans. There are those who own snowshoes and those who prefer snowmobiles. Those who like organic food and those who eat at large Chinese-Mexican fusion buffets. And in parenting there are those who fall into the following three categories, which I call *mainstream*, *alternative*, and *nearly Amish*:

MAINSTREAM	ALTERNATIVE	NEARLY AMISH
Disposable diapers	Cloth diapers	Elimination communication
Formula	Nursing by hospital's schedule	Unrestricted nursing
Crib	Cosleeper	Family bed
Stroller	BabyBjörn	Handmade silk wrap
Circumcise	Circumcise if Jewish	Over my dead body
Placenta in biohazard bin	Placenta planted under oak tree	Placenta dried, ground, and ingested as daily supplement
Cut cord right away	Wait till cord stops pulsing, then cut	Keep cord attached to placenta for three days until it falls away naturally. Carry placenta in knitted bag with Rastafarian color scheme

Gwen and I fall somewhere between the second and third columns, so Gwen decides to nurse. She has done her research and found out why breast is best. Plus, she can simply feel it. We are animals and we (meaning Gwen) make milk for our young. And this milk is best for them in every way. The same body that in some incomprehensible miracle creates life and grows a baby also produces the milk. They come from the same source. They are *literally* made for each other.

Breast milk is beyond science. We have yet to fully understand it, and we will certainly never reproduce its equal in a laboratory. It is a mystery, like quantum physics and black holes and the appeal of Bikram yoga. It is God manifest in the material world. I get a bit fired up about breast milk.

And here are some of the wondrous perks of breasts. I mean, of breast milk.

The first milk that comes out after baby is born is called colostrum. Colostrum contains gentle laxatives that help baby poop out the meconium. It contains probiotics that set up the proper flora in the baby's gastrointestinal tract and is higher in protein than ordinary milk. Colostrum also contains antibodies to protect the newborn against disease. These antibodies set up the infant early on with a healthy immune system. They contain the combined disease prevention protocol of mama. Pretty awesome! Think about that. And when you nurse, if you have a cold, you pass your own antibodies to baby. In this way, I like to imagine that each generation gets stronger.

Every mammal produces colostrum for their babies. It seems so sacred to me, a special bond between mom and newborn baby. In southern India they sell a special sweet cheese made from cow colostrum. When I first read this I literally choked back a vomit, and then I realized that it was no different from cheese made from regular cow milk. New things can seem so scary.

Breastfeeding bonds mama and baby. It is nature's way of saying, "Hey, stay near your baby. She needs you." And there is literally no better soother or TLC than a nice, warm nipple. Visualize this. You've had a tough day of learning to use your fingers. You're frustrated after the fifteenth time you dropped the ring that dangles above your head. You're craving some touch. Well, now, there's that warm soft fleshy mama who smells so good. The warm nipple that fits just perfectly in your mouth. And the milk, oh, the milk, let me tell you! Delicious. And you always fall asleep after drinking it. Ah, sweet ambrosia.

Breast milk is a panacea. It generates hormones in mama that battle baby blues. A few drops heals pink eye. I've seen this first-hand, and it's amazing. Noah had pink eye. Gwen posted this to Facebook and asked for advice (*yes, we get our medical advice from Facebook*). A friend told her to express a few drops of breast milk right into Noah's eye. And that cleared it up. You could see the redness disappearing as in time-lapse photography.

Breast milk also cures chapped nipples and lips and fights baby acne, and the list goes on. I suspect that it could loosen tight lids and finally get my car door to stop squeaking. But Gwen is always so hesitant to try these things.

My friend Jenny was worried that her breasts were not large enough for nursing. All breasts are, by the way, but she was really concerned. This must be some urban legend like getting pregnant from sperm in bath water. But during pregnancy a woman, any woman, gets real big. Jenny did get pregnant and in, like, three months, she went from Mila Kunis to Sofia Vergara, but without the accent.

Breastfeeding is not always easy. Especially at first. What is, though? And, unfortunately, misinformed healthcare providers often jump at this stage to recommend formula. When I brought Noah to Gwen in the hospital after the pediatrician checked his lungs for meconium, Noah had trouble latching. Many babies do, and, in fact, getting a baby to latch right after birth helps set the tone for successful nursing. Gwen struggled for a few minutes and then Wendy came over and showed her a trick to slightly open and untuck Noah's lip. Another good reason to work with a midwife or doula. That created the perfect suction and Noah latched and didn't let go...for two and a half years.

There are hard times. Pain, clogged ducts, infection. For these

Wendy taught Gwen to use cabbage leaves. Seriously. And they worked. More than once, Gwen sent me out to the market for a head of cabbage. She'd take a large leaf and cup it over the affected area. Have you ever heard of the doctrine of signatures? It's the idea that herbs and plants in nature give us clues by looking like what they help. This is amazing. A cross section of carrot looks just like a human eye. A walnut is like a minibrain and contains the fatty acid DHA, which is food for the brain's neurotransmitters. And think about a leaf of cabbage. It looks exactly like a breast. It even has veins and a nipple bump!

It is very rare for a mother not to have enough milk, though this is a common fear and chorus at hospitals and from pediatricians. I imagine they might be getting this from the conventions they attend in Puerto Vallarta when they stand together in mass groups under strong lighting, repeating the phrase "supplement with formula" as the Nestlé CEO shouts at them from the podium.

If your supply seems low, get help. Whatever your problem, be it pain, infection, or simply fear, ask for help. Midwives, doulas, breastfeeding support groups, and La Leche League educators can help. You are not alone. I promise they have seen your problem before, and I promise they will help you.

Chapter 11

Attachment Parenting

Attachment Parenting has been around
as long as there have been mothers and babies.
It is, in fact, only recently that this style of parenting has
needed a name at all, for it is basically the commonsense parenting
we all would do if left to our own healthy resources.

— William and Martha Sears, *The Baby Book*

*N*orthampton is the yoga, holistic health, folk music, and lesbian capital of the United States. Which also means we have more cats per capita than the Lion Kingdom. We have one lesbian and two cats for every man in town. The welcome banner at the Northampton parking garage says, "Welcome to Northampton. Where the coffee is strong, and so are the women."

The Noho crowd loves bumper stickers. My favorite is "I look forward to the day when schools get all the money they need and the military has to run a bake sale to buy a new jet."

I also love the bumper sticker of British suffragist Rebecca West's famous quote, "Feminism is the radical notion that women are people."

I think we attachment parenters need a similar bumper sticker that reads, "Attachment Parenting is the radical notion that babies are people."

Gwen and I, wandering the house in an unslept stupor, would remind ourselves of our personal Attachment Parenting motto, "A baby's wants are his needs." This is true. Babies are pure cause and effect, action and response. They do not plot or manipulate. They simply tell us what they need. Just think how scary it would be to be a tiny person who can't do anything for herself. You'd need your big warm cooing parents to take care of you. And you'd get frustrated trying to let them know the difference between when you are hungry and when you've had a poop. And if they ignored you, you'd get really pissed.

Kevin and Lena, two physics profs at Smith College, were our first friends in town to have kids. They are both scientists, so before they make a decision, they do their research. When they make up their minds, I trust that they have considered all the options. If Lena tells me that coconut oil is best, I need look no further. I have no doubt that she has interpreted the research correctly. Kevin and Lena were the first to turn us on to the "Sears Book."

William Sears is a pediatrician in California who popularized Attachment Parenting. He studied in Boston and Toronto in the 1960s and teaches at the University of California, Irvine. He has written more than thirty books, is the parenting consultant for *Parenting* magazine, and has been a guest on every talk show, including *20/20*, *Good Morning America*, *Oprah*, *CNN*, the *Today* show, *Dateline*, and *Wayne's World*. Okay, not *Wayne's World*, but he's been on a lot of shows.

In his books and talks, Sears lays out seven precepts to Attachment Parenting. Precepts scare me. My mind can turn these into another list of anxiety-producing do's and don'ts. Another list to obsess about, another explanation of how I have failed and why my kids will need some serious therapy. But Sears's list is different. It essentially says: *Trust your baby, trust your parenting instincts, and get support from friends and family.* Which may, indeed, be the very key to Conscious Parenting.

His seven precepts to Attachment Parenting are as follows:

1. *Birth bonding — connect with your baby early.* Take an active role in the birth you want. Educate yourself. Speak openly with your obstetrician, midwife, and/or birth attendants. Be present for the birth.

2. *Read and respond to your baby's cues, that is, cries.* Newborns don't misbehave. They communicate. We just need to watch and listen. And try things. Even if you misunderstand a cue — offering a nurse when all little Jimmy wanted was a cuddle — he'll tell you and you will refine your ability to understand. This is similar to honing your intuition. That is, the best way to cultivate and hone intuition is by listening for and then following intuitions as they arise. As Malcolm Gladwell teaches in his bestseller *Blink,* each time you follow an intuition, your intuition strengthens. This, I'd say, is a great example of what's meant by *follow your parenting instincts.* I love seeing this as a skill that, with practice, I can hone.

    Sears says: "Pick up your baby when he cries. As simple as this sounds, there are many parents who have been told to let their babies cry it out, for the reason that they must not reward 'bad' behavior. But newborns don't misbehave; they just communicate the only way nature allows them to.... A baby whose cries are not answered does not become a 'good' baby; he becomes a discouraged baby."

3. *Breastfeeding.* We've discussed this already. The benefits of breastfeeding are endless. Mom gets happy hormones. Baby gets antibodies. No one has to get up in the

middle of the night and walk across the cold linoleum to mix a bottle.

4. *Babywearing (carrying baby in a sling or carrier)*. Trust your instinct to hold your baby. Sears says carried babies cry less and grow more. And they feel safe and get to snuggle up to you. When I see a baby in a very crowded mall being pushed in a stroller, the baby always looks the way I feel on a roller coaster. "Where am I going? Where's Mom? HELP! Ahhhhh!!!" That dialogue, by the way, is a direct quote from me at age thirty on Disney World's Space Mountain.

   In Northampton, parents favor baby carriers and wraps and are embarrassed by their strollers. There's always a qualifier: "I'd have all three boys in a carrier on my back, but I threw out my SI joint in *chaturanga* last week."

   For a long time, Gwen and I did not use a stroller. And this drove my parents bananas. They'd have purchased us the coveted Bugaboo Donkey stroller in three different colors if we had let them.

   Finally we relented. Noah is heavy and I have hurt my back more than once trying to shift his weight while I was in an awkward position. I bet almost every sling- or wrap-wearing parent has a similar story. We could compare wounds.

   Here's our rule. Okay, it's Gwen's rule. But I follow it. We always carry or wear the boys in crowded areas, but we allow ourselves the pleasure of a stroller on quiet streets or sometimes in the woods.

5. *Bedding close to baby (cosleeping)*. Sears wonders when and why this practice became so controversial. He has

found that because it's so discouraged in the mainstream, lots of families who actually do cosleep don't admit to it. Plus, he reminds us that most babies the world over sleep with their parents. And that we evolved to do so, which makes pretty good sense. Historically, babies left alone would be threatened by predators. I can't imagine that native peoples put their baby to bed in a small cave or teepee nearby before retiring to their own master bedroom.

6. *Balance and boundaries.* Take care of yourself. Put on your own oxygen mask first, as they say. A healthy baby needs a healthy mom and dad.

   Take a night off. Hire a sitter, or call Grandma. Exercise. Eat well. You'll be a better parent when (at least a few of) your own needs are met.

7. *Beware of baby trainers.* Don't be convinced to follow any dogmas. Ignore any advice that counters your parental instincts to nurture your baby. Parent from your intuition and your heart.

That's it right there. Sears's seven Bs of Attachment Parenting. I love that they are not dogma but a call to empowerment. They are a call to wake up to my instinctive parenting wisdom: being alert to each moment, assessing what is needed with clear eyes and an open heart. Intuition. Flexibility. Mindfulness. If nothing else, it's an excuse to keep doing yoga and meditation, now that there's really no time for it.

Chapter 12

Say Good-Bye to Your Luscious Down Comforter

I used my week of leave and have headed back to work. Thankfully, Gwen's folks are staying nearby to help out. No matter how private you are, letting a relative help you after the birth makes all the difference. People are not meant to do this alone.

When I get home from work, I throw on a sling and wear Noah while we eat. Actually, first I accost him with kisses. And he cries. I learn to approach him slowly, but this takes every ounce of discipline I can muster. The feeling builds in my short car ride home and by the time I pull into the driveway, I am ready to jump from the moving car and roll to a stop at his little feet.

Knowing that I will wear him in the sling and be right next to him helps slow me down.

So does knowing that I will spend the night next to him. Gwen and I have decided to cosleep. That means that little baby Noah sleeps in bed with us. Cosleeping brings up a few questions and concerns and sometimes even an angry mob with pitchforks and torches. I'll address each of the concerns in turn.

Question 1: What does that do to your sex life?

Answer: If you are asking this question, you clearly do not have young children. Because, my friend, after birth there ain't much sex for quite some time. Can be six weeks, can be six months. Depends on the circumstances. Don't forget, in birthing, a woman pushes an eight-pound watermelon that has shoulders out of her vagina. So that area can be a bit sore for a time.

And then she's nursing and not sleeping, so there may not be much sex drive. And basically, let's face it, biologically speaking, the point of sex is to create new life, so her body just thinks, "Been there, done that, got that one checked off the list." So her body may not point her in the direction of the lube and handcuffs for a while.

Question 2: Isn't cosleeping dangerous for the baby? Don't people roll over onto their tiny fragile newborns?

Answer: As my friend Kevin aptly puts it, "The humans who roll onto their babies evolved out long ago." Plus, even when you're asleep, you know where things are. I mean, when's the last time you fell out of bed? You could sleep a whole night right on the edge, and you'd never fall out. Your sleeping body/mind somehow knows exactly where it is in relation to its environment.

Now, there are a few caveats. Human beings did not evolve with down comforters. So these are a no-no when cosleeping. Gwen and I had to trade our luscious down comforter and pillows in for boring cotton. I like my bed to be like a big cloud of cozy comfiness, like Brony Smith's bed in her scandalous yoga videos for Equinox Fitness. A down comforter could settle onto a baby's face, block his nose and mouth, and obstruct breathing. But a regular blanket provides no such danger. Even so, most of us keep the blankie a bit lower when we cosleep. This might sound less cozy than tucking it up over your neck and shoulders, but you just wear an extra layer to bed, and having your luscious little bundle cozied next to you trumps the blanket tenfold.

The other caveat is imbibing drugs, alcohol, and even certain prescription medications. These substances can numb a person's sleeping senses and make him a danger to an infant in the bed.

I'm working eight to five (or six) every day. Sleeping next to Noah keeps me feeling connected to him. If he slept in a different room, I'd get two, maybe three, hours a day with him, but sleeping together, we spend twelve or more hours a day near each other. Sometimes I wake up in the middle of the night and just sniff him before falling back to sleep.

(As I edit this manuscript now, a few years after writing this chapter, just thinking of a tiny baby sleeping beautifully right next to me, almost, almost, makes me want to call Gwen and try to convince her to meet up at lunchtime to try for a third.)

Cosleeping has infinite perks. We don't have to wake up in the middle of the night and creep into the nursery to check on Noah's breathing; he's right there with us. The classic mainstream conception of nursing is: baby cries, mom gets up, slides feet into slippers, zombies into nursery, lifts baby from crib, sits in rocker to nurse until baby falls back asleep, returns sleeping baby to crib, zombies back to bed, and sleeps for an hour or two until next waking.

And that's okay. But how's this scenario? Baby is sleeping between mom and dad. Baby is ready to nurse. Baby moves head to the right, finds nipple, and nurses and mom doesn't even wake up. Mom sleeps the whole night and baby just comes in for a snack whenever she wants.

This has happened exactly three times...in history. Okay, so maybe not that scenario so much, but at least baby is already right there when you need to nurse. Plus, studies show that when mama and baby sleep together, they will match each other's sleep cycles.

The baby sleeps better and mom and baby will wake together rather than at unharmonious intervals.

A few times a night Gwen wakes me for a diaper change. That is my job. And I am a diaper-changing machine. She can nurse and roll over and sing to Noah and I won't wake up. But the slightest, quietest, "Brian, diaper change," and I am up. "Gotta make the donuts."

It is amazing how we attune to these things. Take my mom, for instance. My dad snores like a Shop-Vac. I'm not even sure it's legal to snore like he does. But on a sleepover, when a friend and I would sneak downstairs, the slightest, quietest creak of floorboard and she'd be all, "Brian, is that you?" Honestly, I don't even know how she could hear this over my dad's Homer Simpson–like jowl-jiggling growls.

There are times when cosleeping is not the best setup for a family. And I've heard of some pretty funky sleeping arrangements. A friend, Cordelia, spent three years in the jungles of Brazil with Doctors Without Borders and was impressed by how well babies slept swinging in hammocks. So her baby sleeps every night in a baby rocker, the kind that electrically rocks back and forth while playing Pachelbel's Canon.

Lots of folks I know use a cosleeper, a small contraption that attaches to the bed and gives a baby her own space. This is especially useful for parents who fear that they will roll onto their babies. It's a fine plan and I'm all for it, though mostly, in my experience, the baby winds up in bed and the cosleeper winds up holding diapers, mama's water bottle, and a few magazines.

For a few weeks, Gwen tried the Canoe. This is like a very snug hammock that swings from a tight spring attached to a big bicycle hook mounted in the ceiling. When baby stirs, the movement causes the hammock to swing and rock the baby back to sleep. It worked until Noah was six months old and wanted more freedom to move his arms and legs. He'd get frustrated and wouldn't sleep a wink. So we took it down and sold it on Craigslist for half of what we paid. We still have the large red hook in our bedroom ceiling. Visitors probably assume that we are very into Iyengar yoga, Pilates, or some seriously kinky S and M.

Chapter 13

Get Help!

Asiyefunzwa na mamae hufunzwa na ulimwengu.

— Swahili proverb roughly translating to, "It takes a village to raise a child."

Noah is not sleeping well. And therefore neither is Gwen. Sometimes in the middle of the night she growls into her pillow.

The obvious answer is for us to use Cry It Out or its kinder, gentler twin, Ferberizing.

Cry It Out is an approach to getting babies to sleep. It was first proposed by Dr. Emmett Holt in 1895 in *The Care and Feeding of Children*. Interestingly, Holt is often considered the father of pediatric medicine, though I suspect midwives might propose that medical care for children has been around a bit longer. I suspect thousands of years of doctors, shamans, medicine men, witches, and midwives are turning in their graves, saying, "So, what about me? What am I? Chopped liver?"

I always enjoy reading medical pamphlets from the 1800s. To keep a mother's milk supply abundant, Dr. Holt recommends drinking plenty of "milk and gruel." I like the word *gruel*. And, like everyone at that time, Holt was terrified of masturbation. He ends his pamphlet with a discussion of thumb-sucking, nail-biting, bed-wetting, and masturbation, in which he concludes that "masturbation is the most injurious of all these habits, and should be broken up just as early as possible. Children should especially be watched at the time of going to sleep and on first waking. Punishments are of little avail and usually make matters worse. Medical advice should at once be sought." I wonder what he may have meant by medical advice. Castor oil? Circumcision? Miniature chastity belt?

Holt introduces the world to Cry It Out with the following Q and A in the pamphlet:

Q: *How is an infant to be managed that cries from temper or to be indulged?*

A: It should simply be allowed to cry it out. A second struggle is rarely necessary.

To answer the follow-up question, "Is it likely that rupture wilt be caused from [this] crying?" Holt recommends using an abdominal band to prevent said hernia.

Holt popularized Cry It Out in 1895, and it is my theory that the method caused both world wars, twenty and forty years later, when these very pissed-off babies became adults.

Thankfully, ninety years later along came Dr. Richard Ferber to tone things down a bit. Ferber's method, described in his 1986 book *Solve Your Child's Sleep Problems*, recommends that rather than simply abandoning your baby to cry until she stops, as Holt had recommended, we should allow a baby to cry for a designated amount of time before we comfort her. This, Ferber posits, teaches a baby to self-soothe.

Ferber recommends beginning bedtime with nighttime rituals, putting baby in her crib, and then leaving the room to return at progressively increasing intervals to comfort the baby verbally or with a pat. But do not pick up baby.

On the first night of Ferberizing, you return first after three minutes, then after five minutes, and thereafter every ten minutes, until the baby is asleep. When she reawakens later in the night, you repeat the process.

Sometimes this takes days of dogged persistence and of ignoring your parental instincts to comfort your baby.

If I wanted to be convinced to use Ferber's approach, I should not have read the rest of his book. Later, in regard to discipline for older children, Ferber is big on setting limits. What if your five-year-old leaves his room after lights out? Ferber says to set up a gate so she cannot leave: "The gate often becomes a symbol of this change, and the same child who fought the gate initially may now remind you to close it every night." That's exactly what I want. For my child to become most comfortable when incarcerated. To model the Stockholm syndrome.

If the gate does not do the trick and your child topples dressers, remove the dressers. Sometimes it's even necessary to remove everything but a mattress from the room.

I'm always on the lookout for things that posterity will point to and say, "No! Tell me you didn't! How could you?" The way we now look at slavery. And I'm fairly certain that Ferber's limit-setting approach will be one of them. It'll be right up there with the fact that every teenager carries a cell phone in the pocket next to his or her genitals.

Ferber's approach seems like sheer torture to Gwen and me, and we simply can't do it. I suppose we have the luxury of making this choice since Gwen is not back to work yet and since, really, she's so darn tough. I fear that being up so many times in the night would kill me.

Gwen is tired and mighty grumpy, but she believes it is worth it. We won't use Ferber, but surely my large pile of parenting books has something more to offer us in the sleep department. Gwen and I try every holistic and natural solution we can find. We read *The No-Cry Sleep Solution*. Gwen sees midwives and asks parents at La Leche

League meetings. She tries the Canoe. We try ritual and routine. When Noah is one and a half and decides to sleep in his own bed but still wakes up hourly, we rub Gwen's sweat onto his stuffed rabbit so he'll feel like she is always near. No dice. Nothing works to get him to sleep through the night. In all the books and research, we never really find anything that helps.

Now, I must say that in some lucky cases, babies are just happy sleepers and everyone is in bliss. And some moms, when awakened by a baby stirring, roll over, nurse, and fall right back to sleep. Some never even wake up. But not most, and not Gwen. She is a light sleeper. So this is a very rough time. Very rough.

I think the real problem is threefold. First, it's actually not us old folks at age thirty-five or forty who should be doing this. We're supposed to be grandparents. For most of human history, people had kids at, like, age fifteen. When I was fifteen, I could stay up half the night and feel fresh in the morning. I could sleep on a wood floor at a friend's house and wake up to play tackle football. Now my back hurts if I skip one day of yoga. But I see no fix to this issue; I am not advising folks to have babies at age fifteen.

Second, our ancestors probably didn't have to get up early to catch the A Train to Manhattan. And, frankly, they probably didn't have to think very much, let alone design PowerPoint presentations and have engaging water-cooler conversations with the boss. We need government-mandated extended maternity and paternity leave. In Italy a parent gets 80 percent wages paid for five months of leave. And in Denmark, it's a whopping 100 percent for a full year.

The third problem is that we are not meant to do this alone. To live in tiny nuclear groups. Back in the day, you would have nine people from three generations in one house, and everyone would share the labor. My sons love the children's chapter book *Milly-Molly-Mandy*, written in the 1920s by Joyce Lankester Brisley. The main character, Millicent Margaret Amanda, aka Milly-Molly-Mandy, lives at the edge of a small village with her mom and dad and auntie and uncle and grandma and grandpa. And everyone has a role in the household. Father grows vegetables, mother cooks, grandpa sells the produce, grandma knits their woolies, uncle tends the cows and chickens, and auntie sews frocks and cleans house.

It might seem strange that her mother's main job is to cook. Like, what does she do the rest of the day, after heating up the burritos that she bought at Whole Foods? But back then, cooking for a family was a full-time job. She'd bake the bread and prepare the soup stock and ferment the cheese and cure the meat and can the jam. At least all along she could have conversations with adults or ask someone to watch the baby while she bathed or walked to town. Plus, afterward, she could catch a nap because she wasn't also doing the laundry, cleaning the house, and handling the garden. Which is exactly what Gwen was doing. I helped, but I was at work all day, so she did most of it.

These days you have only two adults, and there's way too much to do. To this conundrum, though, there is a solution. Instead of having grandma watch the little ones while she knits, we pay a babysitter. Instead of visiting the village shaman or rabbi with our troubles, we have a weekly session with a psychotherapist. Instead of grandpa and dad shoveling out the walk, we have a large man named Ed with overalls and a snowplow.

I choose to simply think of Jewell the housecleaner as Auntie Jewell, and Rick the lawnmower guy as Uncle Rick.

And I believe that this may very well be the key to a healthy marriage as well. If you can find in your budget an extra $30 a week, try hiring a biweekly housecleaner and a kid down the street to mow the lawn or shovel the walk, and spend the rest on a babysitter so you can get some dinner and have sex, and you'll be back on your honeymoon. You might even save money, realizing that you no longer need your couples' counseling.

Or you can set this up with neighbors as a trade. Share the labor and save the money. You watch Wilma and Ed's baby along with yours for a few hours while they shovel both driveways or mow both lawns. And then next time switch roles. This way you can all nap while the babies nap rather than having to use that time to sneak out to do the chores. You can even ask a neighbor who owns a snow blower for an occasional favor (maybe include some cookies in the deal). The same goes for asking trusted neighbors or friends to babysit. You'd be shocked what folks are willing to do to help people who have little kids.

Gwen and I are working on making these changes, and we've come a long way. But it takes effort. You see, I am Jewish and from the tri-state area of New Jersey, New York, and Connecticut, which means that I have no problem asking for help and even paying people to help me. In Jersey, we have 403 phrases for this. It's like the Eskimos with snow. Gwen, on the other hand, grew up Catholic in Canada, which means she will drop from exhaustion before allowing someone else to cut the grass, clean the house, cure the meat, or can our jam. She is a homesteader. And I respect that. Secretly, I know she is better than me and I want to be more like her.

But, for now, with little kids, I am with Hillary Clinton and the Swahili; it really does take a village to raise a child. And since we no longer live in tribes, we need all the help we can get.

Chapter 14

What Is This, 1850?

*M*y sister and I have an ongoing contest. Whoever seems more natural and hippie-ish gets a point. When I had hay littered about the backseat of my Corolla after hauling a bale to my community garden plot, I got a point. When she and her boyfriend started brewing hard cider from local apples (now famous, by the way, as Citizen Cider), she earned a point. If either of us grew dreadlocks we'd have a lifetime win. Game over. But, in the meantime, when Gwen and I opted for cloth diapers over disposables, we took the cup for the year.

Cloth diapers are superior to disposables in every single way, except convenience. They do not fill the landfill with plastic and with human feces. They are easier on your baby's sensitive skin. They are even far superior in helping little Hazel potty train. More on that later.

But cloth diapers are a pain in the ass. They smell. You have to scrape the poop into the toilet. You have to keep a bin in the bedroom to soak them, and you have to do a lot of laundry. And cloth diapers get stained. They're vile, really.

They are also beautiful and now that we are done with them, I have the fondest memories. I would happily use one as a pillowcase or to wrap my lunch in. What else is so closely associated with your baby? Just thinking of trifolds brings back memories. Memories of sweet, innocent yellow breast milk poop, memories of the boys crawling around the family room.

It's all our friend Jeremiah's fault, really. He first told us about cloth diapers. And actually, we bought our first set of diapers used from Jeremiah for $400. *Four hundred bucks!* And they were stained with his kids' poop. When else have you paid $400 for shit or shit-stained anything? Maybe fertilizer, if you're a farmer; I'll grant you that. But nothing else. When kids are in the picture, all bets are off. Imagine buying a crate of skid-marked adult boxer briefs for $400.

I can't be too pissed at Jeremiah for the price. These things are like gold. Gwen and I are now done with the diapers, and recently, we had a garage sale. We posted an ad on Craigslist: "Kitchen items, used printer, books, kids' toys, baby clothes, and cloth diapers."

We received the usual inquiries from eighty-year-old men named Eustis looking for bottle caps and coffee tins from the 1950s. But apart from that, every single call was about the diapers. People asked us to put certain sizes aside for them. They asked for certain brands. They begged us to reserve them until they could get to us at 7:00 AM. I felt like we were launching a new type of Cabbage Patch doll. One guy at the garage sale bought five pairs and whispered, "Any that you don't sell, give me a call, and I'll give you a good price."

Cloth-diaper buyers constitute a zealous garage sale subculture. I bet there is a thriving brown market on eBay. No pun intended. And, in fact, no one at all, not even once, on the phone or in person, inquired about shit streaks. These, I suppose, are assumed.

Jeremiah taught us his three-step cleaning process:

1. Scrape the poop into the toilet.
2. Soak in a pail with a fifty-fifty water and vinegar mixture.
3. Run them for two cycles in the washing machine with hot water and no soap.

No Whisk or Tide or even Arm & Hammer. Which, of course, explains the excessive streaks in his batch. But I'm all for it. I wouldn't want harsh detergent next to my baby's soft delicate skin, anyway.

Even at $400, cloth diapers are a bargain. From birth through age three, for one baby, you would use approximately seven thousand disposable diapers, which costs $2,000. And that's for the el cheapo Pampers imitation from CVS. If you buy the best disposables for you, your baby, and the environment, say, from Seventh Generation or Earth's Best, you'll be paying upward of $5,000.

There are also gDiapers, which are simply ingenious and I was sure must be another fantastic Google innovation, like Gmail and Google Docs. But it turns out that these diapers were actually invented by Jason and Kimberley Graham-Nye, which explains the name. The Prius of diapers, these are a hybrid of reusable exterior and compostable insert. As with the other earth-friendly disposable options, to diaper your tyke in these, you'll be spending thousands.

Cloth, on the other hand, costs twenty bucks per diaper, which seems insane — a full set could be a down payment on a new houseboat or vacation home. But, this one diaper is worth, like, a hundred disposables. And you'll be saving exactly that many from the trash heap. Plus, you'll also be preventing that much pee and poop from sitting in the landfill, leaching into the water supply and winding up in your kombucha.

Cloth diapers are also healthier for baby. Mainstream disposables often contain dioxin, a toxic chemical associated with reproductive and developmental problems. And those clever little gel blobs inside the diaper that in a feat of science and wonder absorb

113 ounces each contain sodium polyacrylate, which was removed from tampons for its association with toxic shock syndrome.

I even read recently that mainstream disposable diapers, which are made up of plastic polymers, act as insulation and can keep your baby boy's junk (that's a hip word for penis and testicles) too warm, a factor that can lead to infertility.

Which is just way too much for me to be thinking about. My anxiety is peaking right now. I may need to break for some *pranayama*.

Cloth diapers, on the other hand, are made of, well, cloth, so they contain no dioxin or sodium polyacrylate, and they don't over-insulate.

Cloth diapers are also better for the environment. Behind newspapers and beverage containers, disposable diapers take up the third most space in landfills. And each neatly wrapped diaper entombs a nice bit of pee or poop that goes untreated and, as mentioned, ends up in the soil and water.

And here's a perk you may not have even expected. Cloth diapers actually help kids learn to pee and poop in the potty. Disposables soak the wetness away so fast kids don't even know they've peed. But in cloth diapers they can feel it and they ask for a change. They can tell they have peed so they make the connection. "I peed, I feel wet. Maybe I should pee in a potty like mom and dad do." I've seen this with my own kids and with many of our friends' kids as well. It's a beautifully organic process. You can avoid the bribes and gold star charts. Alfie Kohn would be thrilled!

There is only one downside. When you sign on for cloth diapers, you join the cult. You, too, start wandering garage sales looking for used BumGenius, FuzziBunz, OsoCozy, BottomBumpers, TushieSombrero, and AssHat cloth diapers (okay, I made up the last two). You'll talk about your diapers at parties, weighing the pros and cons of trifolds versus flat inserts. And you must decide whether to wash or to hire a service.

In Northampton, we have a service that will pick up your soiled diapers.

On a bicycle.

Seriously. That's how we roll here in Northampton. I'll say it again. People come to your house and pick up your kid's shit. On a bicycle. They will also haul away your trash and recycling to the dump, bring your compost to a farm, and, in January, in a wonder of physics, take away your Christmas tree. On their bicycles. I'm not shitting you.

Chapter 15

My Osteopathic Shaman

*N*oah is one year old. He enjoys torturing Gwen and me by climbing onto the headrest of the couch and walking back and forth like a tightrope walker. One evening, midtightrope, he took a misstep and started falling. As he slid between the wall and the couch, I dove onto the couch to catch him. I got him, but I landed in a very awkward position, arms extended, and I couldn't get the leverage to lift him.

I yelled to Gwen for backup. She rushed into the room and got hold of him. She thought I was going to stand up to let her get into a good position, but instead, after having grown up with way too many action films, I rolled dramatically off the couch. Which is precisely where Gwen swung her leg. Hard. And she is Canadian. These people are like stone, so darn strong and hard. It's how they survive the winters. That and plugging in their cars. So the ball of her foot slammed into the bridge of my nose. I actually heard a crack in my head.

To be fair, I do have a prominent nose. And this was by no means the first time it had taken a wallop. Maybe it's large enough to have its own gravitational field that pulls feet and volleyballs and small children to it. Plus, this runs in my family. You could read my grandpa's nose like the rings of a tree. "Ah, yes, that's from 1921 when I was kicked by a horse while bringing grain to the mill. And this bump here is from '35 when Munyo, a gentile, was drunk and accidentally head-butted me in a tavern."

Enter the kombucha. I had recently discovered the stuff. Kombucha is a fermented drink made from a very nasty-looking, mucousy mushroom. A bit of the mushroom floats in every batch and looks exactly like snot floating in soda. But I love it, and since it's fermented it has the slightest alcohol content and makes me a bit tipsy. In fact, I have to avoid kombucha because whenever I get my hands on it, I just start chugging. Which is exactly what I did in a natural foods café the day after Gwen broke my nose. I had just chugged a pint of kombucha to ease my nose pain and I was enjoying the giddy high.

But kombucha also has cleansing properties, so too much at once can cause the body to dump toxins and make you sick. So there I was, nose broken, drunk on kombucha, and getting a cold, when a friend's mom walked by and asked how I was. I told her about my nose, my kombucha high, and my impending cold. She, as we tend to do in Northampton, referred me to her current favorite holistic practitioner — in this case an osteopathic shaman named Edmund.

Three days later, I showed up for my appointment. At the center of Edmund's office was an altar to his ancestors, replete with giant eagle feather, Brazilian drum, and stones from the Amazon. In a sterile American hospital, you'd be tackled to the floor by security for even thinking about wild animal feathers.

Edmund began with a prayer. Then he placed his hands on my head and moved his fingers around very slightly... for about twenty minutes. Then he was done. He told me there was a small crack in my nose and that during our session my body had released strains from the break.

And actually I felt much, much better. The best, in fact, that I had felt since before Gwen had kicked my head. Better, even, than that.

I have continued to see Edmund as needed over the years. After Noah accidentally tackled me in a parking lot while I was holding baby Benji and, to avoid landing on either boy, I was forced to go down headfirst onto the pavement, I saw Edmund. When, during rumpus time, Benji kneed me between the eyes, I saw Edmund.

And each time I leave Edmund's office feeling twenty again.

So I'm a convert. In fact, now I, too, have an altar to my ancestors in my office. I believe, in fact, that it's partially responsible for helping me get this book deal.

So what's the moral of this tale? It is this. I think the world needs more kombucha, more altars to our ancestors, and plenty of osteopathic shamans to help us release strains after our kids accidentally tackle, trip, knee, kick, elbow, and head-butt us.

Chapter 16

The Vulcan Baby Grip

My own preference,
if I had the good fortune to have another son,
would be to leave his little penis alone.

— Dr. Benjamin Spock

Dr. Benjamin Spock is not played by Leonard Nimoy. I know this. Yet, when I first saw his photo on a book jacket, I was shocked to see a white-haired gentleman. I guess I still expected pointy ears and jet-black hair.

Dr. Spock's sixty-year-old tome, *Baby and Child Care,* sat on my bedside table for months before I dove in. The 1950s seemed like the dark ages to me. I pictured his world in black-and-white. Plus, for some reason I had thought that Dr. Benjamin Spock was a bad dude. A villain in the genre of holistic parenting. I associated him with hitting kids. I think this came from a Woody Woodpecker cartoon from my youth. The cartoon, as I remember it, showed a mother opening a parenting book that contained not pages full of advice but instead a compartment holding a hairbrush with which to spank kids. For some reason I remember the book title being something like *A Parent's Guide to Discipline, by Dr. Spock.*

But I must be remembering incorrectly, because it turns out that Dr. Spock was a righteous dude. The message of his book is to honor children, to listen to them, and to treat them as individuals.

As mentioned earlier, Spock's main message to parents, especially to mothers, was, "Trust yourself. You know more than you think you do." He was all about empowering them! And this was in the 1950s, when people were totally repressed. I've seen *Mad Men*. I know all about these folks.

Spock himself was an ardent political activist, later protesting the Vietnam War. He was arrested numerous times for civil disobedience. Not only that, but at points in his life he meditated twice daily, ate a macrobiotic diet, and practiced yoga. I love this man!

Apparently Spock's stance on Vietnam was unpopular with supporters of the war, so they attacked and attempted to defame him. This might explain the Woody Woodpecker reference. And apparently their campaign was successful. In fact, the only other thing I remember hearing about Spock is that his own son committed suicide — a fact that was supposed to unequivocally invalidate Spock's work. But the fact is that Spock's son did not commit suicide. His two sons are alive and well.

The Spock story gets better and better. He was slated to be Dr. Martin Luther King Jr.'s vice presidential running mate in the 1968 election. And he actually ran for president in the 1972 election under the People's Party. His platform: free medical care, the immediate withdrawal of all American troops from foreign countries, a guaranteed minimum income for families, and the legalization of abortion, homosexuality, and marijuana! Amazing!

Spock's parenting mission was to counter the prevailing behaviorist notions of the day. Parents believed that babies should not be held or coddled, since doing so would breed needy, spoiled individuals, unable to deal with the harsh world. So Spock was basically the foil to Holt's 1896 *Cry It Out*.

If Spock were here today, he'd be a full-on attachment parenter. He'd be wearing Prana-brand yoga pants and hanging out with Rodney Yee. He and Alfie Kohn would be mixing it up at tea shops, and he'd be playing in the mud with Larry Cohen. He'd be traveling the Attachment Parenting speaking circuit and offering workshops at Kripalu, Omega, and Esalen. His kids would be breastfed, coslept, uncircumcised, sleeping on sheepskin, and wearing organic wool, and Spock himself would be following his parenting intuition.

In Spock's own words, "The more people have studied different methods of bringing up children, the more they have come to the conclusion that what good mothers and fathers instinctively feel like doing for their babies is the best after all."

This is similar to Dr. Sears's message, and I feel sure it must be true. If not, if we have lost this instinctive ability that all animals have to care for their young, then bring on the glaciers and comets, because our epoch is done.

Like that of Dr. Sears, Spock's message frees me up. It invites me to relax, get conscious, and follow my own parenting instincts. It calms my anxiety and reminds me that if I go inward to find answers, and if I try my best, even when I'm overwhelmed and unsure, I'm probably doing just fine.

Chapter 17

The Perfect Parent

The twentieth-century philosopher Fred Rogers said, "My hunch is that if we allow ourselves to give who we really are to the children in our care, we will in some way inspire cartwheels in their hearts." Then he put on his sweater and changed into sneakers.

Maybe I can come clean to Noah and the world that this parenting thing is pretty darn challenging. That I have no idea what to do quite a bit of the time.

Another modern philosopher, Louis Szekely, albeit from a different school of philosophy than Mr. Rogers, has his own take on this: "It's hard having kids because it's boring.... They read *Clifford the Big Red Dog* to you at a rate of fifty minutes a page and you have to sit there and be horribly proud and bored at the same time." Szekely, also known as Louis C. K., certainly speaks his mind.

We're not superhuman or infallible. And our kids will wear us down and find this out. When we've got nothing left, they will ask for one more story. While we're having sex for the first time in seven weeks, they will wake up and call for a glass of water. And they will call us on our hypocrisies.

So I'd like to stop trying to be perfect. Instead, I'd like to model being human. To learn from my mistakes. To apologize when I mess up. My plan: forgive myself and move on. Kids are so incredibly dynamic. Today I can start being the parent I want to be. And if today does not go quite right, I can forgive myself again and start fresh tomorrow.

Last week, I was at an eye exam for Noah. The doctor was kind of a jerk. He wanted to put drops in Noah's eyes, which I can accept. But apparently he had not read Dr. Spock or Dr. Sears. And he certainly was not versed in Larry Cohen's very excellent Playful Parenting approach. This doctor would have made a very fine navy admiral. But as a pediatric optometrist, I'd say he was ill suited.

He was frustrated that Noah, age two, did not want to sit still for the drops. Which is weird. Was Noah his first patient? Maybe pediatric medicine was a new career for him, perhaps after retiring from the NYPD vice squad.

So the doctor commanded me to hold Noah down while he put in the drops. Noah was crying wildly. I was caught off guard by the doc's order, so I did it. I held Noah down against his will while the doctor put in the drops.

Afterward, Noah cried some more. But then he moved on pretty easily, thrilled to play with the toys in the waiting room while his eyes dilated.

I, on the other hand, felt terrible. I was sure I could have found a less violent way to get the drops in. I had overpowered Noah physically and felt I had betrayed him. I was beating myself up. But then a friend reminded me that my job as a parent is not to model being perfect but to model being human and compassionate and forgiving.

When we got home, I apologized to Noah and told him that I would never do that again. Which I think is valuable. I don't need to model getting everything right. That would be too neurotic. It's okay to mess up. I just need to model taking responsibility, apologizing for my mistakes, and forgiving myself.

After all, kids learn from what we tell them, sure. But even more, they learn from what we do. So if I can do this, if I can forgive myself, well, then, Noah will likely learn to forgive himself.

And that would truly be something worth passing along.

Chapter 18

Punished by Rewards

The deepest impulse in the human self
is to be lovingly related to people....
A loving human being is not produced by exhortations,
rules, and threats. Love...emerges in children
when it is poured into them.

— Huston Smith, *The Illustrated World's Religions*

Noah is no longer a tiny baby. We need new advice. *His wants are his needs* is no longer enough. What about discipline? What do we do when he throws his applesauce against the kitchen wall? How the heck do we get him to put on his pants? We find help in Alfie Kohn, author of *Unconditional Parenting*.

I am hesitant to let my dad know that I am reading Alfie Kohn's book, let alone that I am applying his theories to my parenting, for two reasons. First, Kohn's name makes him sound Jewish, and he's not. Which will be so disappointing to my dad. When I meet a new friend, this is always my father's first question: "Is he Jewish?" In fact, my dad seems no longer able to encode for any friends who are not Jewish. He flawlessly remembers every Jewish friend's name but is at a complete loss for all others, calling every one of them Rudy, regardless of their name or even gender.

The second problem, and this is a big one, is that, ultimately, Kohn's message closely resembles that of (cover my grandma's ears) ...Jesus. Yes, the Christ. The ultimate Christian. Gentile ground zero.

You see, Jesus felt completely loved by his dad. Unconditionally. And as a result he was able to fully love his disciples. With no restrictions, small print, withholding, or strings. He wasn't trying to get something from them, and he wasn't trying to elicit their compliance or get them to cooperate. He simply loved them fully. Exactly as they were.

And in feeling loved, the disciples became free. Free of insecurity. Free of baggage. Free of worry. Free to be themselves. Free to act from their truest impulses, from their hearts. Even when persecuted, even when tortured. There are historical accounts of the disciples in peace or even rapture while being killed or tortured. Why? Because they felt deeply and truly loved.

And this is exactly the message of Alfie Kohn. That we as parents must love our kids unconditionally, with no restrictions, small print, withholding, or strings. Deeply and truly. We must simply love them fully. Our job is to make sure they feel loved for who they are, not for what they do or how they behave or how pretty their artwork is or because they do what we tell them to. Our job is to make our love, in a word, unconditional.

Now that I have exposed this scandal, I hope my dad can still accept, even love, Mr. Kohn. Don't forget, after all, that Jesus himself was a nice Jewish man. Perhaps the nicest one ever. He didn't beat up any Philistines, turn his staff into a viper, or circumcise his grown son. Nope, he just loved and loved some more.

Kohn points out that most parenting approaches ask the question, "How do we get our kids to do this or that?" Which makes sense. Getting our kids to do what we want will certainly make it easier to get on their snow boots and get out the door on time in the morning. But, says Kohn, we are asking the wrong question. The real issue is not how can I get them to do what I want, but rather, "How can I help them become who I want them to be?" Happy. Self-confident. Successful. Ethical. Compassionate. Which, really, is why they go to school or ballet or Spanish class and why we are trying to get out the door in the first place.

Asking how to get kids to comply, to get their boots on and get out the door, is myopic. It gets us out the door in the morning, but at what cost? This approach, focusing on getting compliance, leads to a "doing to" approach of punishments, rewards, and bribes. "If you don't get ready now, I'm going to [threat]," or "If you get your boots on, we'll get [reward] after school."

And the studies show, Alfie says, that doing things to kids to get them to obey does not in any way foster kids who are happy, self-confident, successful, ethical, and compassionate. In fact, it does the opposite. It simply fosters kids who learn how to earn the biscuit and avoid punishment, like well-trained poodles. Punishments, rewards, and bribes can result in compliance, but studies show that they make kids self-centered — what do I need to do to get what I want?

I was not always a Kohn fan. In fact, until Noah was two, I had never heard of him. Gwen found him first.

One night, after Noah's bedtime, Gwen and I are hanging out on the couch. She taps the book she's reading and tells me, "This says that praising kids for doing a good job actually builds insecurity. It makes them seek the praise rather than a job well done."

I can tell she's referring to me and the way I speak to Noah.

Generally, telling your partner that you disagree with how he or she parents results in, wait, what's that phrase...oh, yeah, a shit storm.

And, of course, that's because I know she's right. I do praise Noah too much. I want to build a temple every time he poops. My tribe does this; the Jewish people dote on their children. Who else has an actual word for "bursting with pleasure and pride, especially regarding one's family"?

Plus, I was raised on praise. Really, my whole generation was.

It's not my parents' or your parents' fault. It was just the times. And now I am addicted to it.

Here's an example. Last week Noah was home sick. In the morning he and I stretched out on his bed and colored together. He made a nature scene, and I drew a house with flowers and a shining sun.

I went to public school, so my art development pretty much clipped at third grade. I have been drawing this same house for thirty years. And this one was a great version. Noah got new beeswax block crayons for his birthday. They have four different surfaces, each of which produces a different effect. He has learned to employ these different surfaces, and he taught me.

So I made a gorgeous version of my picture and literally couldn't wait for Gwen to get home so I could show her. But she is not my grandma and she did not kvell. Plus, I am thirty-six, so I suppose it's simply less impressive now.

I was disappointed. Even mad.

Which is really pretty nuts. I know this.

I think I have an unhealthy relationship to approval in general. Last year, after my first memoir came out, when I'd wake up each morning, I'd head straight to my iPhone to check my Amazon ranking. And each morning I'd be either elated and on top of the world or a total wreck. I can tell you that deriving one's sense of self-worth from Amazon rankings is an even worse plan than deriving it from a spouse's opinion of a crayon-colored house.

I don't want to model being neurotic and needy. I don't want to teach Noah to derive his self-worth from the opinions of others. I will try to stop praising Noah (and checking Amazon every morning).

But how? I start by reading Alfie's book.

Kohn says, "If we want kids to be concerned for others, we would never praise them for sharing. Studies find that kids praised for sharing are less helpful because they do it for the biscuit." If you give kids prizes for reading, they will lose interest in the books. What you are rewarded for becomes less appealing.

Kohn says positive reinforcement is conditional love. Praise says, "Only when you jump through my hoops will I give you what you want." Kids must not learn to see our reaction as the point.

My generation is victim to this. I remember using the Systems 80 machine in elementary school. This device, believe it or not, is modeled directly on Skinner's box — the one that Harvard professor B. F. Skinner designed to give cheese to rats for pushing a lever. It turns out, in fact, that the theory that most influenced child rearing and education in the United States in the past hundred years was originally based on Skinner's work with training rats.

Skinner demonstrated that a rat who gets a treat from pressing a lever will repeatedly press the lever. He then extended this finding to humans, espousing "operant conditioning" in raising children, that is, using rewards and punishments to elicit desired behavior. If a child produces the correct behavior, she gets a reward. If not, she gets a punishment. Just like a rat. Eventually they (the children and the rats) behave as you want them to.

All this is why I was so hurt that Gwen ignored my crayon picture. Even as I drew it, I was fantasizing about who might praise it. I just wish my editor would let me include it in the appendix. I know you'd like it.

Seeking praise warps what I'm really feeling. It trumps my actual impulses. I've spent the past twenty years attempting to deprogram this. All day, I ask myself, "What am I really feeling? What do I truly believe?" Not, "What will garner praise?" but "What do I really feel? What do I really care about?" Which is especially useful now as I attempt to tune in to my parenting intuition and instincts.

Just last week, I was in a meeting with Noah's nursery school teacher, and halfway through I realized that I was more focused on what she thought of me than I was on helping Noah.

Alfie's books say that to avoiding passing this habit along to our kids, we need to use evaluation-free statements such as, "You put your shoes on by yourself" or "You did it." These statements say we've noticed without heaping on judgment. Kohn even addresses the artwork. What is it with kids and artwork? "If your child draws a picture, you might provide feedback — not judgment — about what you noticed: 'This mountain is huge!' or 'Boy, you sure used a lot of purple today!'"

So the idea is to note actions or specifics: "Look at Emily's face! She seems pretty happy now that you gave her some of your snack." Praise would emphasize how I feel about Noah rather than showing Noah how Emily feels.

Plus, Alfie advises, rather than saying, "Good job!" we should ask questions. "Why tell him what part of his drawing impressed you when you can ask him what he likes best about it?" or ask, "How did you figure out how to make the feet the right size?" This, says Kohn, will likely feed his interest in drawing. Saying "Good job!" might actually have exactly the opposite effect.

I'm ready to give it a try.

For some reason Noah has decided to make a chart showing the Hebrew letters and their English equivalents. That's just the kind of thing he likes to do in his spare time. Remember, he's only two, so I see this and immediately start, "This is amazing! Gwen come and look at…"

Stop. I steel myself. I stand a little taller. "Noah, ah, *you did it.* Look at how this chart, er, ah…there are letters."

I am about as smooth as Steve Carell in *The Office.*

I try again. "Noah," I say, "how did you think to make a chart like this?" He tells me all about it, beaming. Not because I'm pleased, but because he's pleased and enjoying himself. Cool. Maybe I can actually do this. You know, I think I did a pretty good job with that. Oh, boy, maybe Gwen saw me…d'oh!

By the way, yes, Kohn is antipraise, but be careful here. This is not advice to completely avoid praise. It is wonderful and essential to let our kids know how much we adore and love them. We can acknowledge their achievements and character. It's just that these must not be associated with our approval or love. Our love must be unconditional and unchanging.

So loving unconditionally does not mean that you become an unfeeling automaton. And it certainly does not mean that you hold back when you are overcome with the need to smooch your kid and give him hugs and nibbles and a big ol' belly bizurt. Not at all. That would be sad.

I had a friend whose parents were intellectuals living in Cambridge in the 1970s, the kind of liberals who would later show her the exact Cambridge row house in which she had been conceived. They understood that praise can strip a kid of motivation. That kids can start to work not for enjoyment but for the praise. "For the biscuit," as Alfie says. So they did not praise her. Ever. They never commented on her report card. Or her gymnastics moves. Or her beautiful hair.

They surely had thoughts and feelings, but they never, ever shared them. And she grew up. And she was self-directed. And she did things because she wanted to, not to please others. And she did things she enjoyed.

But she felt unloved. Literally. I know this because she used to say things like, "I feel unloved."

So I should adore my kids but not use praise as a judgment or as a tool to get them to do what I want. If I am also not using punishments to teach them not to throw their applesauce against the wall, what do I do? How do I get my kids to do what I need them to do? Like wearing underwear at the kitchen table. Is that asking so much? Or just once to help put on their snow boots? Even just to point their toes while I pull on the boots.

Alfie's answer: We should really see our kids and respond from there. He gives the following example. You put little Esmeralda to bed. Two minutes later, she pops out of her room for a drink or to pee or because she's scared or because she wants a snack or one more cuddle. Again. And again.

Instead of rewarding her for staying in bed or punishing her for leaving her room, look at the situation and ask why she's getting out of bed. Really look. Not only at her behavior. Look underneath. Ask why? Why is Esmeralda not staying in bed? Is she hungry? Not tired? Scared of a monster? Stressed about school? Wanting more time with Mom and Dad?

Each of these calls for a different course of action, a different parenting opportunity. We can address the underlying issue. More than just applying a Band-Aid, we can guide, help, and really make a difference in the lives of our children. It's about being conscious and taking children seriously. Having a relationship with them.

Kohn tells a story about a girl who dumps her snacks on the floor. Her dad says, "Put them back in the bag and bring the bag to the kitchen table."

The girl is adamant. "No!"

Dad is about to shout when he thinks to ask, "Why not?"

The girl answers, "Because I want to eat them."

Aha, problem solved. Dad simply explains, "You can still eat them after putting them in the bag; I just want to keep the living room clean."

Kohn states, "Perhaps when your child doesn't do what you're demanding, the problem is not with the child, but with what it is you're demanding....Why does the only place in the world that is truly a child's own have to be maintained according to the parent's standards?" Before we search for a clever way to get kids to do what we want, we should reflect for a moment on the value of our request. Why does Billy have to keep his room up to our specifications?

I love this one. Especially, I think, because my whole mission is to cultivate my intuition and live from that place of inner wisdom. If we want this for our kids, we can help them cultivate it by honoring, when appropriate, their own inner knowing.

I'm not suggesting cake for dinner, but if there are peas and carrots on the plate and Noah loves the peas but hates the carrots, why not honor that? This is not him acting out or being willful. Perhaps his body is telling him what it needs and wants. Listen, and I might stave off a rash from a carrot allergy. Or not. So what? Let him off the hook. Why does he need to eat the carrots?

This also comes up in my house because, as you know, I was raised by wolves (by Jews in New Jersey, actually, but to a Canadian it might as well have been wolves), so I love when Noah eats with his hands. To me, this seems primal and like it connects him to his food. Metal silverware seems so proper and disconnected. So when Noah is scooping up his scrambled eggs and Gwen calls for his fork, I side with him. I think manners are a nice tool to have mastered in case the queen comes calling, but at home, I think, Noah can eat with his fingers.

Okay, so let's put this all together, shall we? Kohn sums up Unconditional Parenting with the following suggestions:

1. *Work* with *kids rather than do* to *them*. When Billy throws his toy, see this not simply as an infraction that demands consequences but as a problem to be solved. Why is Billy throwing the toy? See his behavior as a parenting moment. An opportunity to help him.

2. *Take children seriously*. Treat their ideas and intuitions with respect. They may know better than we do what they want to eat, who they want to play with, and whether they are sleepy. You don't want your kids to

feel that it's only okay to care about or get upset about the things that Mom and Dad care about.

3. *Attribute to kids the best possible motives, consistent with the facts.* Kohn says children form beliefs about their motives based in part on their parents' assumptions about their motives. We can help kids develop good values by treating them as though they already have these values. They come to believe this about themselves and then live by it.

4. *We have to say no so frequently, that when we can say yes, we should.* Is it okay for your child to choose to sleep on the floor? To sit backward on her chair during dinner? To trim her own bangs? Maybe it is.

5. *Don't be in a hurry.* Tweak the schedule when possible to avoid having to impose your will on your kids. Things stay a lot more relaxed when you're not in a rush. Can you move bath time? Wake up ten minutes earlier? Head to the door to put on boots a few minutes earlier? "Plus," says Kohn, "as the cliché goes, kids grow up so fast, and before you know it you'll ask where all the time went. So take the time to savor the now with your kids."

I agree, of course. Still, this last one is hard to hear. It's a heel-on-toe situation begging to happen.

I'm determined to integrate Kohn's insights into my parenting. I certainly don't want Noah to feel addicted to praise. And I want him to feel that I'm on his team. That he's got a pit crew in me and Gwen.

I called upon Kohn just this morning. Gwen and I were at Noah's playgroup. We were watching a friend's baby, and I needed to change the baby's diaper. I scooped her up and started to walk away from the group, leaving Gwen and Noah. Noah started freaking out. I was about to shush him when I paused. I looked at him, at me, at the moment. He is jealous that I'm walking away with a baby. I reach out my hand, "Noah, would you come along and help me change Sienna's diaper?"

He was thrilled to help out. Problem solved. Tantrum averted.

Alfie's advice will be my personal Zen Kohn. An invaluable tool in the Conscious Parenting playbook.

And what about our original query, the applesauce on the wall? Now that we are Kohn experts, let's ponder WWAD. What would Alfie do?

I believe he'd recommend that rather than attempting to change or control Noah, I change the environment. That I turn Noah's chair or engage him while he eats or switch to a different spoon or ask myself whether maybe Noah doesn't like applesauce. Or maybe he'd just tell me to get out a sponge, wash the wall, and let it go. That some mess and chaos is simply part of the deal. To quote Kohn, "If you really are looking for a house of peace and quiet, you may have wanted to choose tropical fish instead of children."

Chapter 19

The Christmas Dreidel

I'm glad to be Jewish. At least I hope it gives this book a leg up. Think about it. Many of the bestselling parenting books come from the tribe.

Playful Parenting's Lawrence Cohen? Jewish.

How to Talk So Kids Will Listen's Adele Faber? Jewish.

What to Expect's Heidi Murkoff? Definitely.

The Happiest Baby on the Block's Dr. Harvey Karp? Absolutely.

What about Blossom turned Big Banger turned author of *Beyond the Sling*, Mayim Bialik? One hundred percent. And she's religious.

And *Unconditional Parenting*'s Alfie Kohn? Dang it, I'm still reeling from that one. Don't tell my dad.

And what of Dr. Emmett Holt, father of *Cry It Out*? No way. Please! Not a Jewish bone in that man's body.

Actually, truth be told, since I married Gwen, I consider myself half-Jewish and half-Christian. Our family celebrates both Christmas and Hanukkah. So at two years old, Noah doesn't really know the differences or distinguish between them. Last month when we went to Northampton's annual Santa's Workshop and Noah sat on

Santa's lap, to the question, "And what would you like for Christmas?" Noah confidently replied, "A *very* big dreidel."

Santa didn't even nod. He just looked perplexed, like maybe someone was messing with him.

Hanukkah had already passed, so I had to scour the town for a really big dreidel. I saw one in the window display of a vintage apparel store, but they weren't willing to part with the display. I tried everywhere I could think of. No one had a really big dreidel. Finally, in my fifth toy store, I found the biggest dreidel I had ever seen. It was translucent and opened so you could stuff it with loot, like the Jewish version of a Christmas stocking.

On Christmas morning, Noah was thrilled with the dreidel. For, like, ten minutes. Then it was meaningless to him. It doesn't spin well and soon the plastic cracked anyway.

My side of the family is Woody Allen to Gwen's Annie Hall. My parents are constantly commenting on how Noah eats. Like Howard Cosell calling a Yankee game. Play by play. "Oh, Susan, look at Noah eat that rice. He's ready for his next spoonful. Oh, it's a pleasure to watch." And Noah has always been a "great eater." If you are not Jewish, you might wonder, "What is a great eater? And how can such a person be two years old?"

We like our progeny to eat. A lot. Maybe we're just happy to have food after three thousand years of fleeing persecution. And it's not just my parents. I, too, can watch Noah eat like you stare at a fire when camping. Mesmerized and delighted.

Three thousand years of persecution has other effects, too. Like whenever a teacher gave me a B on an essay, my parents would invariably say, "*Oh*, I just *knew* he was anti-Semitic."

And if you tell your Jewish grandparents that you are considering a Christmas tree this year, "You know, just to fit in," every Jewish grandparent will say exactly the same thing. They will say, "Oy! Six million, Brian! *Six*! *Million*!"

Jews are fiercely loyal to and trusting of the tribe. I remember, as a kid, I was in a hotel once in Acapulco. We were there because my father was speaking at an accounting convention. I was very proud of him. We had just checked in and I watched a Jewish guy from our tour trade dollars for pesos with a shady-looking character in a coat closet. The guy was leaning against a wall in the shadows and smoking a cigarette. If I were a director setting up a shady character, this is exactly how I'd have blocked the scene. He was the Mexican equivalent of Al Pacino in *Godfather III*. Except that he wore a yarmulke. Afterward, I asked the man who was with our tour, "How did you know you could trust him?"

"Did you see his yarmulke?" the man replied.

Maybe he's right. Let's be honest. The yarmulke does tone down the gangster look a bit. I know Jewish thugs in the Lower East Side of Manhattan might disagree, but how thuggish can you look with a kippah on your head? Add some tefillin, a tallis, and tzitzit, and there's no way I'm buying it. Who's the toughest guy you can think of? Maybe Bruce Lee or Chuck Norris? Notorious BIG, Daniel Craig, or Jean-Claude Van Damme? Okay, visualize your guy. He's looking mean. Now, simply place a yarmulke on his head. What happened? Suddenly he smiles and softens a bit, right? He goes from being tough and mean to kindly, if a bit dorky. Suddenly he is very good at math and maybe lettered in varsity chess. He eats corned beef (the kosher kind) and matzo ball soup. No one looks mean while slurping matzo ball soup.

And I know exactly what my father will say to this. He will remind me of the many times that Israel has whupped some serious ass in a weeklong war. To this I have no retort. The Israelis are tough. There's no denying it. They have to be to put up with all that heat and sand and hummus.

If there is another thing at which Jews excel, it is, as mentioned earlier, doting on their children and grandchildren. To my people, nothing matters more. And I think this can be the nonjudgmental kind of praise. The one that makes kids feel loved for who they are, not what they do. I recall one Passover when I was nine years old and learning to Hula-Hoop. I was terrible at it, as I was, until I found yoga, at anything that required a body. But I stood in front of my grandparents and gave the hoop a turn. I swiveled my hips and got maybe three revolutions before the hoop dropped to the carpet. But my four tiny Jewish grandparents, sitting huddled together on the couch, clapped and cheered with gusto, as if I had just announced my admission into Harvard Medical School or eaten an entire pastrami sandwich. And they'd have done this no matter how many times the hoop spun. They just loved being with me, unconditionally, no matter what I did.

I don't attend synagogue much these days. But, still, I consider myself Jewish. There's no doubt of that. And it's more than the latkes, potato kugel, and hamentaschen that I make for my boys. I am Jewish not in a strictly religious sense but in the deep appreciation and awe of love and family and children that my dad and mom and grandparents have instilled in me. It is this sense of Judaism that I most aspire to pass along to my own children.

Chapter 20

Kids' Yoga

Noah is taking a kids' yoga class with lots of other two-year-olds. It's supercute. They pretend to be animals and crawl around the room and hold postures and have imaginary adventures.

But, little kids, I'm convinced, don't really need yoga.

Older kids and teens, by the way, are a whole different story. They need yoga. Reimagine your teenage years with yoga. Seriously. Picture yourself at age sixteen. What are you wearing? How are you standing? Now insert yoga. You're more grounded in your body. You have self-assurance. You stand tall. You're able to identify what really matters in life. Everything from the boundaries in your relationships to your skin is clearer.

But little kids, I think, don't need yoga. You can do cobra or tree or revolved triangle with them, and it will be fun. They are so cute bending and twisting. I love doing sun salutations with Noah. But, really, *we're* the ones who need the yoga. Our kids need to eat less sugar and to frolic in the woods more.

I need yoga to control my fear that Noah will be eaten by a bear or that the sweaty guy on the elevator is going to grab him and run. Or to deal with the panic when he disappears for three seconds behind the microbrewed soap display at Whole Foods.

I do yoga to stretch and to manage stress — neither of which kids need to do — and on a deeper, more spiritual level, I do yoga to open my energetic channels and allow for growth and transformation. And to live my truth, my dharma. But kids are already doing this. I do yoga to become more like them.

I remember teaching a toddler yoga class and being frustrated that the kids wouldn't do what I wanted. They were giggling and playing. I wanted them to be obsessive, perfectionistic, and neurotic like me.

I can, however, let my yoga make me more relaxed and present, like them. I can let it open my mind so that I see my kids as they are, not as I imagine they should be. I can let it open my heart so that I love my kids as they are, not as I imagine they should be.

We need the yoga. Let them frolic.

Chapter 21

Hypnobirthing

As a kid, I watched a lot of TV. Way too much. Which led to certain misconceptions. I believed that Snickers really satisfies. I thought it might be good, clean fun to be stranded on an uncharted desert isle. And I found great wisdom in the words of Mr. and Mrs. Brady.

Similarly, before Noah's birth, everything I knew about labor and delivery came from the screen: A woman is at home. Her water breaks. She remains relatively calm. The husband panics and hastily packs a suitcase, clothes sticking out as he fastens the clasp. Cut to the delivery room. The woman is pushing, screaming in pain and, between contractions, threatening the man with death.

But it does not have to be like this. There is another way.

And that way is called hypnobirthing.

Why do I mention this?

Because Noah is almost three and is now sleeping through the night and Gwen has more energy. She laughs sometimes. She seems to like me again. And she has a sex drive.

So what do we do? Against all reason, we do it all over again.

The idea germinated while we were out for my birthday at a hibachi restaurant with our friends Jon and Adeline. We met Jon and Adeline in our birthing class aboard the chelation machines. Both our kids are now almost three years old and we are feeling revived. Adeline first mentions the idea. Next thing we're all headed home, eager to conceive.

Again, we get pregnant very quickly. My birthday is in October, and Benji is born nine and a half months later in July. Jon and Adeline wind up only two months behind us.

Since Noah's birth, Gwen has learned of hypnobirthing. This is the best-kept secret in birthing. Just as corporations supposedly thwarted the electric car and the United States railway system, I'm convinced there is a conspiracy here, probably headed by the company with the patent on epidurals.

Hypnobirthing is basically the idea that a birthing mama can relax her body and let her baby come out naturally and virtually pain-free. The name comes from the idea of using self-*hypnosis* to relax during *birthing*.

One of the midwives we had met three years earlier when Gwen was pregnant with Noah advocated hypnobirthing. We looked at her the way my parents stared at us when we announced that Noah would be born at home. I remember she said, "When a cat goes into labor, her body is relaxed, she moans a bit and her litter is born. It can be the same for humans."

Which is basically hypnobirthing. I'd still be skeptical, had I not seen Gwen actually do it.

Hypnobirthers think of birth as a natural physiological process, not as a medical emergency that demands a hospital with doctors in scrubs and masks. They believe that the body knows exactly how to birth, just as it knows how to breathe and pee and digest and conceive and nurse. They contend that it is our very fear of birthing that tenses the body and causes the pain. They say that this fear triggers a fight-or-flight response, causing blood to leave the torso and pelvis, that is, uterus, and go to the arms and legs.

The solution? Examining, exposing, and shedding our fear. Creating a comfortable, safe birthing environment. Trusting the body. Training in the art of relaxation. Learning breathing exercises. These are the practices of hypnobirthing.

All this makes good sense. It's sort of a no-brainer. You are pushing a baby through your cervix and vagina. This is no time for clenched muscles. And fear is the biggest tightener there is. Think of a terrified person. Her face goes pale from lack of blood. So, too, does the uterus. Literally. Midwives report a white uterus in cases of extreme fear. A tense uterus is clenched and unable to relax and do its job.

In applying this practice, Gwen is not alone. Lots of folks have taken up hypnobirthing. A 2006 compilation of five existing studies demonstrated that women who used hypnobirthing techniques were half as likely to need painkiller medication and one-third as likely to use an epidural.

Gwen borrowed a CD from a friend and practiced the self-hypnosis techniques, including visualization, relaxation, and deep-breathing exercises. I think she had a leg up after ten years of guided relaxation and breathing exercises during yoga classes. You literally get better at relaxing as you practice.

The breathing exercises include Sleep Breathing (a deeply relaxing breath), Slow Breathing (to use during contractions, which hypnobirthers call uterine surges), and Birth Breathing (for the final stage of labor).

Sleep Breathing relaxes the body before birth and is used between contractions to restore relaxation. It is basically abdominal breathing with a slow, relaxed exhalation. That is, in Sleep Breathing you allow your belly slowly to rise and fall with each inhalation and exhalation. Of course, you're not really breathing with your belly;

expanding the belly lengthens the diaphragm, which expands the lungs for a full, deep breath.

Slow Breathing also involves taking an abdominal breath, but much, um, slower. You practice this breath during each uterine surge (contraction) by very slowly inhaling and pushing your belly out like a balloon and then very slowly exhaling and allowing the belly to relax. When the uterus surges, the muscles rise. Actively expanding the belly in Slow Breathing assists and supports the work of the uterus so that the surge is more effective. The opposite, fighting the surge and holding the breath, opposes the body's work, reduces efficiency, increases pain, and stalls the process.

The third technique, Birth Breathing, is used during the final stage of labor, the stage some folks call pushing. Hypnobirthers call this phase "breathing down your baby."

Rather than pushing, you relax and allow your body to birth your baby.

In her seminal book on the topic, Marie Mongan teaches the technique this way: "Take in a short, but deep, breath through your nose and direct the energy of that breath to the lower back of your throat and down through your body behind your baby in the form of a 'J' — down and forward. Allow all of the muscles of your vaginal area to open as though you were letting the breath out through them or moving your bowels."

I like her "moving your bowels" analogy, and I can absolutely understand all this. When I relax my pelvis and wait till my body is ready, glory happens. But, when, on the other hand, I force things and push with all my might (exactly as birthers do in the movies), I am rarely satisfied. And if something startles me or I tense up, forget about today's poop. It's old news.

To this end, Mongan describes, "The best place to practice [Birth Breathing] is on the toilet as you are moving your bowels."

Even if you're not pregnant, you can experience the success of this approach firsthand. Give it a shot. Prepare beforehand with some relaxing abdominal breathing. Incorporate a visualization or guided relaxation, if you know one. Then progress to the potty for some Birth Breathing.

This practice might revolutionize not only the way you birth.

Chapter 22

Never Argue with a Woman in Labor

We were actually planning for Benji to be born at a hospital about twenty minutes from our house. We were planning this until, in a prenatal session three weeks before Gwen's due date, the hospital's midwife asked if Gwen wanted to give birthing at home another try.

After Gwen's six-day labor with Noah and our hasty transport to the hospital, we had become wary of another home birth. But, at the midwife's suggestion, Gwen lit up. She hadn't realized it, but this was exactly what she wanted.

We scramble to interview home-birth midwives. Cecilia, the apprentice from Noah's birth, is now a midwife and part of a practice in a nearby town. We decide to work with her. We had already hired Ananda, a local doula, to help out both during and after the birth. At a hospital she would communicate with staff on our behalf. At home, as well as assisting with the birth itself, she can play with Noah, cook a meal, fold laundry, or mow the lawn — whatever needs doing.

We have one meeting with the midwives and one meeting with Ananda. Ananda asks us to delineate our birth plan — how we see it all going down. We throw up our hands. Last time our birth plan had not included a six-day labor. Some things, we've learned, cannot be predicted.

The night after Gwen's due date, I am in the den working on my laptop. With the calm of a second-timer, Gwen walks in to let me know: "The contractions started a few minutes ago. I'm going to bed."

"Okay, get some sleep. I'll be in soon." No drama; we are old hands at this. I plan to finish up my emails and make arrangements to be out of touch for a few days. Soon I head to bed. But Gwen stops me at the door. "Let's walk a bit. Things are picking up." We pace the hallway for a few minutes.

Gwen rubs her belly, surprised by the intensity of the contractions, and says, "I think you should call the doula."

I call the doula. Whereas midwives focus primarily on the birth, a doula's role is to support the mama in all phases of birth—to rub her back, get ice pops, and offer inspiring Marianne Williamson quotes. Ananda says she'll be over in forty minutes.

Gwen and I walk for a few more minutes.

Somewhere between the bathroom and the kitchen, Gwen leans over, palms the wall, and says, "I think you should call the midwives."

I figure the midwives will just send us back to bed, but I call. Cecilia says she'll come by.

We walk a few more steps and Gwen says, "Go to the kitchen. Look in the menu drawer for the green folder that Ananda gave us. Find the sheet on rapid birth and read it."

Unless you are a midwife, a doctor, or a big fan of YouTube instructional birth videos, you do not want your wife to send you to the menu drawer to study up on rapid birth.

I find the folder. I read it. It mentions blankets, towels, and a hot water bottle. It might as well be dated 1823 and include recommendations for a good leeching. But frankly, I don't believe we are that close, anyway, so I'm not too nervous. Noah took six days to crawl the half foot of the birth canal, and today we are only an hour into our first night.

While I am in the kitchen reading, Gwen relocates to squatting in the den. She calls out to let me know that her water has just broken. I rush in, leaving the folder behind. Gwen is down onto all fours, swaying her body and using her hypnobirthing breathing.

She's in the zone and seems oblivious to my presence, except when she looks over her shoulder to ask, "Can you see anything?"

"Like what?" I don't know what she means.

"Like a baby."

I almost laugh. I don't see anything.

That moment the midwife arrives. Thankfully I had had the foresight to unlock the front door. Okay, Gwen had had the foresight to unlock the front door — she told me to do it, right after she told me to call the midwives.

Cecilia finds us in the den and kneels down next to Gwen. She takes one look and says, "I can see his hair. This baby is coming out."

Fifty-seven seconds later Benjamin is crowning.

A minute after that, he is in Gwen's arms. I hold him while Gwen births the placenta.

I had gone to bed at 11:00 PM, and Benjamin was born at 11:52. He beat his big brother, Noah, by about five days and twenty-two hours. When Gwen had sent me to read about rapid birth, I doubted her, but I hadn't argued. I knew rule number two: *Never argue with a woman in labor*, but apparently I did not know rule number one: *Never, ever, doubt a woman in labor*. She knows exactly what to do.

I had read the rapid-birth instructions, but I'm glad our midwife made it. The instructions said to have something soft for the baby to land on, but I didn't imagine that he would actually fall out. I'd only really ever seen two births: three years earlier, when Noah was born, and a calf in the film *City Slickers*. I really can't say if I would have caught Benjamin. I like to think *yes*, but I just don't know that I would have seen him coming. Plus, he was so slippery.

Twenty minutes later, the rest of the team of midwives and the doula show up.

I post a photo on Facebook. In minutes we had twenty-six comments. Though my sister makes a good point. "Wait, I just got an email from you an hour ago about your new book. Did you email while Gwen was in the middle of active labor?" Amazingly, I had not.

Benji nurses and the midwives look him over. We all finally go to bed at three in the morning. At six-thirty Noah wakes up and calls me in, as usual, with, "Dada, I'm awake!" I sit on his bed and tell him, "Noah, sweetie, during the night, your new little baby brother came out of Mama's belly."

His eyes go wide. He smiles.

I say, "Let's go into the other bedroom to meet him."

Noah leads the way. He gets up onto the bed and coos to our little baby.

"His name is Benji," I say.

"Hello, Benji. I love you," Noah says.

Noah is three and never without his Little Sweet Monkey stuffed animal, whom he has *never, ever* shared with anyone. He places Little Sweet Monkey onto Benji's tiny chest. Gwen and I cry.

"Can I hold him?"

Noah holds his baby brother for the first time.

And then business as usual. Potty. Breakfast. By seven-thirty we are on the driveway drawing with chalk. At 9:00 AM, Noah and I are at a local mini–golf course for a round of putt-putt.

❧

It is very unusual for a hospital midwife to recommend a home birth. So I wonder if she had a feeling. An intuition. Because, really, she saved us. There's no way we would have made it to the hospital. Benjamin surely would have been born on the side of the highway.

And perhaps Gwen knew, too. Once the hospital midwife suggested it, even colored by her previous epic six-day home labor, Gwen knew a home birth was best.

The moral of the story?

Always trust a pregnant mama. She truly does know best.

Chapter 23

Greased Lightning

I hate car seats. For every reason. I hate installing them, having to wrestle the seat belts and clips into place. I'm sweating now just visualizing it. The way you have to bend awkwardly over the car seat and reach and reach and jam the clips into the LATCH anchors, pushing crumbs and lint under your fingernails. And then to tighten the straps by pulling and slightly jumping up to make sure you get a strong enough tug. I bump my head on the dry-cleaning hook every time. And I especially hate the clip that goes over the headrest; it's always slightly too short and yet the strap is, like, sixteen feet long, so I have to tuck all the excess behind the seat.

And when you have to move a car seat, there's the petri dish of Trader Joe's Os and dust bunnies and pennies and rotting banana that festers underneath.

Sweating and hurting my back and cleaning the rotting putty beneath are actually the easy part. At least these are tangible. I can do something about them. The worst part is the anxiety; have I installed it correctly? When I rock the seat side to side does it move less than one inch? Is the seat substantially reclined but not more than 45 degrees? Will my actions result in the death of my child?

In New Jersey, now, you're supposed to go to the fire department to have your handiwork checked out before bringing a baby home from the hospital. Yet when I was a kid, we didn't even have car seats.

I vividly recall a trip with my family in 1979 to Kutcher's, a Jewish resort in the Catskill Mountains.

My sister Julie is three years old, my brother Larry is eleven, and I am seven. We are in my dad's Lincoln Town Car on the Taconic State Parkway. The *Grease* soundtrack is in the tape deck. Larry is wearing orthodontic headgear and singing as best he can. I have a perfect bowl cut and imitate big brother Larry's every move. Julie is talking to her favorite Barbie.

All three of us are in some crazy seventies PJs...and none of us are wearing seat belts. Furthermore, there are no car seats, booster seats, or child safety devices of any kind in our car or, likely, in any other cars on the Taconic. Julie, Larry, and I are cuddled in a puppy pile in the backseat, tickling, snoozing, wrestling, and snacking on Raisin Bran right out of the box.

Back then no one wore seat belts. And car seats, as we know them, had only recently been invented in the 1960s and had been rejected by parents as extravagant and unnecessary. Manufacturers petitioned the government to mandate the seats, and in the late 1970s states began to adapt laws to require them. Even as of 1984 only half of automobile passengers under the age of four were in a child seat.

Nowadays, Julie and I would be in car seats, and the scene would be different. Nowhere near as homey and comfortable. We'd each be strapped in. Separate, discrete, and upright.

Obviously, I know we need car seats, I guess. Or maybe they are just another superfluous safety measure of our overly anxious society. Couldn't we just hold babies and let kids cuddle in the backseat? Remember the *way back* of your mom's station wagon? There were definitely no seat belts there. We were like projectile missiles waiting to be deployed in case of the slightest accident. Yet, I don't actually remember anybody ever getting hurt. Or did they?

I looked into this, and as you may have guessed, no one is going to give me the go-ahead to ditch the car seats. That would be a lawsuit waiting to happen. According to the Centers for Disease Control, "Placing children in age- and size-appropriate car seats and booster seats reduces serious and fatal injuries by more than half." And from the National Highway Traffic Safety Administration, "Child safety seats reduce the risk of death in passenger cars by 71% for infants, and by 54% for toddlers ages 1 to 4 years."

In fact, in 2011 there were 18,000 fewer traffic fatalities than in 1979. That's a 36 percent reduction. And that's especially impressive, considering that in the same time period, car travel doubled. Currently, you can expect one death for every hundred million miles traveled. Which is actually not too bad. You could drive four thousand times around the equator before getting snuffed out.

No matter. I still hate the seats.

At least they have come a long way. The first car seats were bags with a drawstring that attached to the backseat. This kept little baby Ezekiel from rolling onto the floor or falling out of your Model T but made him curiously resemble a large bagged ham.

Really I hate car seats because Benji does. And because I am sad that Gwen's dad, Gary, whom we call Pop, is sick. Two weeks before Gwen's due date, Pop's cancer takes a bad turn and we need to make the eight-hour drive to say good-bye.

We can't bear to strap tiny newborn Benji into a seat for eight hours, so we wait two weeks. Even so, strapping a two-week-old into a car seat breaks our hearts. And is sheer torture for all of us.

Some kids seem okay with car seats, and others don't. Benji is in the second camp. Every twenty minutes he cries and we stop on the side of the highway for a diaper change and a nurse. After five hours we are only halfway, so we stop at a hotel for the night.

Imagine, instead, though, if little Benji could have been sleeping and nursing right on Gwen's lap. His experience in the car would have been completely different. And rather than Gwen being tortured and powerless to soothe him, he'd be right on her lap and they'd be soothing each other.

We didn't make it in time, and Gwen's dad never got to meet Benji. Which is so sad. I know he'd have liked to, and I know that he would have been touched. Benji is his spitting image.

We miss you, Pop.

Chapter 24

Kids' Korner

*G*wen knows when a tumble down the stairs needs a trip to the ER and when it needs a kiss. She knows about brushing teeth and how many layers are appropriate for a 47-degree day. She knows at what age it's safe for a child to sleep with a pillow. She knows when to transition from high chair to booster seat and how many strawberries you can eat before feeling sick.

Without Gwen's sage counsel, my kids would be wearing shorts in the winter and fleece-lined pants in the spring. How does she remember that Noah should wear jeans that fasten with a button only on weekends? And how do you tell when it's hat weather? I am in awe of the constant sorting of clothes by season and as they grow.

Also, what is safe for babies to chew on and when is a toddler ready to play with small toys? And, right now, I need to know how to intervene when another child snatches Noah's toy.

This last scenario is one of the most awkward for me. I'm off from work today and giving Gwen some time at home alone with Benji, so I bring Noah to the Northampton Kids' Korner. This is the basement of a church that has been transformed into a wonderland for children. There is an arts room and a sand table and a large area with mats and a place to ride tricycles.

First we play in the art area. I am in awe of Noah's ability, positive that he will join the lineage of great masters. I hang Noah's finger painting on a clothesline to dry, and we proceed to the toy pit. A few minutes in, Noah takes a toy from another child. No problem, I give it back.

But then a kid takes Noah's toy.

What can I do here? I mean this kid actually *took* Noah's toy.

So I take it back, too. I try to smile and nod and be gentle, but even so, I can feel the moms in the room eyeing me for a swipe with their diaper bags.

Gwen would have handled this much better.

Chapter 25

Operation Meditation

*I*t's 5:00 AM. I have to pee very badly. And I'd like to go meditate. Someone else would simply get out of bed, pee, and blithely head off to their cushion.

Not me.

To do this, I must pull off a CIA operation.

I must remove the covers, inch by inch — in the dead of night our comforter sounds like a crinkly bag of potato chips. I must crawl to the edge of the bed (our bed is pinned against the wall to make room for Benji's changing table). I must step off, and in the pitch-black, follow the border of the bed frame.

I must round the corner of the bed, where someone who designed our bed has very cruelly placed a jutting protuberance at exactly shin height. At five in the morning I forget this every time. I must stifle my cries. Power through the pain. Eyes tearing, I round the corner and toe the balance-beam width between Benji's changing table and our bed, ever careful, ninja-like, to step lightly.

I am almost out. But now I face my greatest challenge. The small distance between me and the door, maybe five feet, is a minefield of creaky floorboards. Gwen has them memorized. For some reason I do not. At first I pause to consider my options, and then I panic, sprinting the short distance to the door. My feet land extraheavy, and the floorboards creak like mad...yet no one awakens. Hashtag grateful.

On the way out, I shut the door in one motion, careful that it does not squeak, promising to myself that today is the day I will remember to oil the hinges.

Failure in this operation is not an option. Benji is not sleeping more than two hours at a stretch. Neither, therefore, is Gwen. She is grumpy. I *must* not wake her or Benji.

If stage one of OPERATION MEDITATION goes well, I can leave the room with Benji and Gwen still asleep. Now I'm in the hallway. I must pass Noah's doorway without him stirring. He can sense me. I must cloak my scent, my very energy signature. Any stirrings, and he will roll over and groggily say something like, "Dad, lie with me." Which is lovely. Truly. But it's not why I am out of bed. I am heading to my cushion to meditate. Plus, Noah's bed is two inches too short for me. So I cannot stretch out my legs and I won't fall asleep. I will lie there listening to him sleep. Content, but wishing I were meditating or asleep in my own bed.

Alternatively, he could wake up and be alert for the day. Unacceptable. Waking at five to cuddle or meditate is one thing. But art projects and Monopoly are another.

Before I can meditate I must pee. Meditation cannot happen otherwise. The bathroom is opposite Noah's room. I shut his door. Do I also shut the bathroom door and risk a squeak? This one is a judgment call. More art than science. Today I leave it open.

I lift the toilet seat. I pee. To minimize noise, I aim just above the border of the water and the porcelain. Thirty-eight years of standing pees have trained me for this moment. I execute it flawlessly and lower the seat without a clank.

At this point I consider heading back to the lion's den, back to my cozy flannel sheets. This is madness. Gwen and Benji are certain to stir.

Don't do it, I thought-scream at myself as I turn left out of the bathroom. Past Noah's room. Down the hallway. Into my bedroom. Over the creaky floorboards. Around the bed frame. I climb in. Under the crinkly comforter. Ahh. I close my eyes.

Benji stirs.

I am in big trouble.

Chapter 26

Elimination Communication

/t seems just, well, barbaric. Which it is, and let's face it, that's a good thing. The opposite, being civilized, comes with all kinds of problems.

Gwen's friend has loaned her Ingrid Bauer's book *Diaper Free: The Gentle Wisdom of Natural Infant Hygiene.* An unfortunate subtitle, but a fine book. Bauer is credited with coining the term *elimination communication.* Another unfortunate phrase. Bauer posits that babies give cues to when they will poop and pee, and if we learn their cues, we can hold them over the ground, toilet, sink, or bathtub and avoid diapers altogether.

Gwen read the book and is intrigued. It was not really a hard sell; she had nearly been using this approach already with Noah. Since Noah used cloth diapers, he could feel when he was wet, so he reacted, and we could tell. Plus, Gwen noticed that baby Noah pooped at around the same time every morning, so when he was six months old, we bought a potty and started sitting him on it every morning. We were unintentional ECers.

So with Benji she starts right away. We watch for his cues.

Gwen sees that he pees after every nurse. So she holds him in the traditional EC position over the sink, and he pees. (My apologies to any houseguests — for example, Matty Oestreicher — to whom I forget to mention this and whose toothbrushes have fallen into the sink.)

Peeing into a sink may seem odd. But pause for a moment and try, instead, to think of peeing into a diaper as odd. It's not a huge stretch. To practice EC, you have to watch for cues and really get to know your child. You have to attune and be mindful — the perfect practice for any parenting yogi.

Devout elimination communication adherents insist that, in order for this stuff to work, we must practice 24/7, full-time. Which is, obviously, impossible for most folks, who work and can't be around their babies all day to watch for a pre-poop grunt. But I disagree with the staunch EC set; I say do it when you can. Save a few diapers in the evenings and on the weekend. Where's the downside?

In other countries, EC is not such a big deal. In certain African, South American, and Asian cultures, you don't need to read books to learn the signals. They are pretty obvious. You are wearing baby in a sling on your back. Baby squirms. Now you have poop running down your back and legs. Next time you'll remember.

Of course, sometimes there are misses, but by age two, Benji is completely diaper-free and in cute little training undies. Think of all the money we saved. A win-win for us and for the environment.

For our wool carpet in the family room, not so much.

Chapter 27

Brown Bear, Brown Bear, What Do You See?

Noah has just figured out that I have hair on my body and that he doesn't. A developmental landmark, to be sure. Unfortunately, though, his fascination is not so much with my legs, arms, chest, or even beard. He is consumed by the fact that, amazingly, he has no hair down below — on that part of Michelangelo's David that all kids stare at — and I do.

Which is fine. Except that kids have no filters. They will say anything. They don't know that it's funnier to point out your fart at home than it is at the salon. At nursery school pickup, they'll tell their teacher that you didn't wash your hands in the bathroom, or they'll ask you loudly if a woman with a bit of a mustache is a man.

Eight years ago, before I was a parent, my four-year-old nephew shouted angrily at me in a public men's bathroom, "Stop sticking your finger into my tushie!" (I was not, though perhaps I was wiping a bit too thoroughly.)

So now Noah demands a viewing and a comparison at every possible opportunity. I don't believe in making any bodily parts or processes taboo. For example, when Benji wants to inspect the goods before we dump his potty, I say absolutely. (I do draw the line when he wants to use it as Play-Doh.) So when Noah wants to view my hairy David, I go with it.

This came up recently at the Eric Carle Museum of Picture Book Art in Amherst. Noah loves the bathrooms there — not only are the walls tiled with images from Carle's classic *Brown Bear, Brown Bear, What Do You See?* but the urinals are etched with flies AND they have the cutest little minitoilets for the under-seven set.

We were in a hallway crowded with parents and kids headed to the craft room when Noah realized he had to pee. Already excited about a trip to this bathroom to search for the blue horse tile, it hit Noah that he'd also have a chance to... "Daddy, I have to pee, and I want to see your hairy penis!" In his jubilation, he lingered on the last two words, so it sounded like "hairyyy peeeeeniiiiis."

Noah's shrieking glee drew the full attention of the museum's throngs of crafting parents and tots. All I could do was nod, smile, and offer a curt wave.

Chapter 28

Get Me a Beer

Sometimes I do what I want to do.
The rest of the time, I do what I have to.

— Cicero the slave, *Gladiator*

A few years ago, when Noah was two years old, we were at our friend Hugo's house for a party. In this particular group of friends, Gwen and I were the first to have kids, and we had not been out with the group in a while.

At first I was thrown. I didn't know what to make of it. This was not a birthday party, there were no balloons, and I saw no paid entertainer.

There were maybe twenty people at the party. And they just sat around and told stories and joked and talked to one another. And get this, they went to the bathroom whenever they felt like it. And they said funny things to one another, not to distract and stave off a meltdown, but just for the fun of it.

Weird, right?

I did not get to participate in the merriment. Why? Because my son was two and very curious and because people without children have the wackiest shit on their floors. Like samurai swords waiting to be wall mounted, and expensive acoustic guitars, and souvenir Swarovski crystal statues their mothers bought in Austria, and piles and piles of books and CDs. So I was very busy chasing Noah and wrestling samurai swords, tangled guitar strings, and priceless crystals from his tiny clutches.

And here's the real rub. Benji is now one, and Noah is four, and I have no time. Last weekend we got together with friends who mentioned that they had been cleaning their house all day. Gwen and I were dumbfounded. How could they clean while their kids were at home? For us this is simply not an option. The boys seem to require our full attention, from waking till bedtime. So, now that I have two children, I can't for the life of me figure out how I felt so darn busy with only one. What the heck was I doing while Gwen nursed? Did I just sit and watch, awaiting my next task?

Which makes me wonder if Nadya Suleman, mother to fourteen children, would look at me and say, "You *lucky, selfish bastard*! Look at you, eating every day and having solid bowel movements. Man, to have only two kids, well, now, that would be something."

Lately Gwen is busy with Benji at night, so I am on Noah duty. Last night he woke up at 2:30 AM and called me in. He needed a drink of water. I got him one and went back to bed.

Ten minutes later he called me in. He had to pee. I took him to the potty and went back to bed.

Ten minutes later his head hurt. I brought him into bed with me.

I fell back to sleep instantly, but he poked me a few minutes later. He couldn't sleep.

I got up to get his water bottle, gave him another drink, and instantly fell back to sleep.

A few minutes later he poked me. He thought he had peed in the bed. I felt around. "No pee," I told him, but he insisted. I took him to the potty again and realized that his shirt was in fact a bit wet around the collar. He must have drooled or been sweating and thought the wetness was pee.

We went back to bed.

He woke me. He couldn't fall asleep and his head hurt.

My mom, who was visiting, heard all this and suggested Tylenol. I felt Noah's head. He seemed hot. And clearly he was uncomfortable, so for the sanity of everyone, I agreed. (Ordinarily Gwen and I reserve this kind of allopathic medicine for dire illnesses and teething that will not respond to amber necklaces, homeopathic chamomile, clove oil poultices, and eye of newt.) I got up, again, and gave Noah the children's Tylenol.

At this point, it's 4:45 AM. I fell back to sleep and did not hear from him again. I had been mostly up from 2:30 to 4:45 with at least nine back-and-forths to his room, the kitchen, and the bathroom.

At 6:30 he wakes me again. I figure he'll have a full-blown cold now.

He does not. He is chipper and fit as a fiddle, ready to pull me out of bed and do mazes before breakfast. Should I be angry or thrilled that he's not sick?

I ask for two more minutes. He says he'll wait on the couch.

Five minutes later, I get up, head to the couch, and draw some mazes.

Chapter 29

It's Not Personal

Benji (age two): "I'm going to lick the wall."
Me (age forty): "Benji, please do not lick the wall."

Kids will point out to the world that you have hair on your penis. They will innocently note your most sensitive character flaws. And they will say things they don't quite mean. Recently, Gwen has gone back to work part-time after years at home with our boys. Noah couldn't be happier with the extra Daddy time, but for Benji it's an adjustment.

This past Sunday was our first full day without Gwen. Noah and I were setting up a puppet show when I realized that Benji was no longer in the den. Last I had seen, he was arranging his toy farm animals inside a fence.

I look around the house. He isn't in the breezeway playing with his toy car ramp. He is not in Noah's room having a peek at his brother's things.

I find him in our bedroom, blankie tucked around his legs. He is trying to open a tube of Weleda skin cream that Gwen uses on his hands and face when he gets eczema. I sit down next to him.

"Do you want help with that?"

A very tiny, "Yes."

I unscrew the lid, squeeze a blop onto his knuckles, and gently massage it in. I squeeze another blop onto my finger and massage his chin and cheeks. Benji purrs, bathing in the loving touch.

The sun is shining through the window, warming us. Benji and I are cozy and in love, connected, staring into each other's faces.

"I love you, Benji," I whisper.

He smiles, soaking it in, basking in it.

And then he looks me right in the eyes, beaming, his tiny face alight, as he says, "I love...Mama."

But it's not personal. I think right now, for Benji, "I love Mama" is the most powerful phrase he can utter. It's an ode to love. A magical incantation. It's like Papa Smurf saying, "Boy, that Brian Leaf, he's so Smurfy."

Although, really, who knows, because right after that, still gazing into my eyes, he continues, "And I like goats and some hay."

Later that afternoon, Benji is on the potty and asks me, "Why doesn't Mama have a penis?"

Who knows what's stored in these brains of ours, because without even thinking, I say, "Boys have a penis and girls have a vagina." I didn't even know the *Kindergarten Cop* quote was still in there.

Benji is pensive.

I figure it might be helpful to review, so I ask, "What about Uncle Larry — is he a boy or a girl?"

Benji thinks for a moment and says, "Boy."

"Right, and he has a penis. What about Grandpa Manny, boy or girl?"

Benji: "Girl."

Me: "No, he's a boy. He has a penis."

I decide to loop back to Benji's original question, so I ask, "So what about Mama, boy or girl?"

Benji: "Girl."

Benji smiles, excited he got it right, and adds, "So I will call her a vagina!"

Me (very nervous, waving my hands): "No, no, no, she *has* a vagina, so she's called a *girl*. Don't call her a vagina."

He nods. Thankfully, I think he gets it.

Close call.

Chapter 30

Playful Parenting

Play is often talked about as if it were a relief
from serious learning. But for children play is serious learning.
Play is really the work of childhood.

— Mr. Rogers

I feel that Dr. William Sears and I have become old friends. Like a
psychotherapist and client who start to have lunch together.

Or maybe more like a doctor and a needy patient.

We spend many happy evenings together on the couch as Dr.
Sears advises me from within the pages of our dog-eared copy of *The
Baby Book*. He's the first one who mentioned the words *Attachment
Parenting*. He taught me why babies cry and when to worry about
a rash. He taught me to keep the Tupperware in the bottom kitchen
drawer so Noah can empty and refill it while Gwen or I cook. And
he even showed me the birds and bees of postpartum life. I like to
think of him as an honorary grandparent in our house.

But then, when Noah turned just two, Sears got up from the
couch and left me scared and alone. No more checking the mighty
Sears bible for signs of the croup. No more helpful tips on play.

For a few days we were lost. Our small village no longer had its
shaman. What to do? Gwen, ever resourceful, turned to the litera-
ture and finally found guidance in Lawrence Cohen.

Larry Cohen is a bit of a jackass. He prides himself on it. And he's also a genius. Cohen is like Mud Man, a guy I met at a renaissance fair who has a PhD in early-medieval studies, specializing in play. Translation: seventeen weekends a year he drives to renaissance fairs, covers himself in mud, and makes children laugh. He believes society has grown too serious and needs a swift kick in the funny bone. Larry Cohen agrees.

In his wonderful book *Playful Parenting*, Cohen posits that, you guessed it, we should encourage our kids to play and that we should get right down there on the floor with them. Cohen says that kids work out their feelings through play and that we can help. When little Billy kicks you, he is working out a feeling of some sort, and it's more helpful for you to engage him than to shut him down.

How do you do this when your urge is to send him to his room, yell at him, or turn and walk away? Engage by dramatically saying, "OHHH, NOOOO! Your kick has awoken the love monster!" And then chase him down and tackle him with hugs and kisses.

Cohen believes that all misbehavior is really just a matter of disconnection. Kids want to be connected, and play reestablishes and strengthens this connection.

Plus, Cohen notes that a huge number of so-called behavior problems would be solved overnight if all children had a safe, fun place in which to play and run around until they were tired.

Cohen's approach is like energy work or Aikido. Rather than blocking the energy that wants to flow toward completion and resolution, you encourage and channel the flow and allow the block to break up. Maybe Billy is angry or jealous or feeling sad or hurt, but in any of these cases, the connection with a loving parent will help the feelings process and move toward resolution. After the play, little Billy might feel complete and happily move on, or he might open up and talk about a troubling day at school, but the play and connection will always more effectively help him get there than would scolding, tension, and isolation.

Here is a summary of Cohen's principles:

1. *Get on the floor.* Get involved. Play on your kids' level, literally and figuratively.

2. *Follow the giggles.* Cohen says, "If something makes your child giggle, then you do it again" — except for forced tickling. Cohen is a professional joker, but he's very serious about this. And I totally agree. There's nothing worse than forced tickling. It's really just one step away from needing to call Child Protective Services.

3. *Roughhouse.* Wrestle. Get physical. Be safe, obviously, but have at it. In my house, we call it Rumpus Time and say it like this: "Get ready to *Rumpuuuuus!*" Ever since Noah was old enough to hold up his own head, he and I have been getting into it on our king-size bed.

   I'm pretty sure this is how WWF wrestling was invented. Noah likes to step back and hurl his whole body onto mine. As soon as Benji was old enough, he joined in. It was a sad but proud day for me when they first kicked me out of the match.

   Of course, sometimes things get out of hand. Usually these are things instigated by me. I get overcome with my love for these little critters and I want to bite them. Which I can't, because then they'd bite me back. Which is actually not a problem, except that they also bite Gwen and that *is* a problem. For some strange reason she does not like to be bitten. I think it's a past-life thing; maybe she was eaten by a wolf in the wilds of Canada.

   Noah's favorite Rumpus Time game is from the

book *Pete's a Pizza*. Cohen would love this book. The main character, Pete, is looking sad. His dad wants to help. He decides he'd like some pizza. First he kneads Pete. Then he spreads the sauce and cheese, adds the pepperoni, and puts the pizza in the oven to bake. Then the pizza runs away right before dad takes a bite.

4. *Reverse the roles.* Start a game with, "Now I'll be the child and you be the parent." This allows kids to be in charge and feel empowered and build confidence. But be prepared; are you ready to see how Johnny sees you? You might learn something.

5. *Learn to love the games you hate.* Ask your kids to fight and pretend to be fascinated, giving a comical play-by-play. This lessens the charge.

    Cohen's advice: "Are you having battles with your children over bedtime? Play bedtime. Having battles over dessert? Play dinnertime.... [And] instead of one more round of 'You have to get dressed, right now!' try saying, 'There's only one rule: You can't wear one red shoe and one black shoe!' and see what happens."

6. *Accept children's strong feelings.* Cohen says, "Playful Parenting involves expecting and accepting strong feelings as well as little frustrations.... These emotions are at the root of most of the so-called behavior problems that so exasperate parents.... If we just accept the feelings and let them flow, they don't cause half as much fuss. And after the tears are really done, everyone feels better." Translation: Sometimes it's better to hold your child or sit compassionately nearby as she has a big cry

than it is to try to calm her down or solve her problem. Just be there for your kids. I'd say this is equally true for adults.

I love this stuff and use it nearly every day. For example, lately, Gwen holds in her pee and refuses to go potty. She'll dance in place, squirming and noodling, holding in her pee and refusing to go potty, until eventually she pees in her pants. It's a big problem.

(Okay, it's not actually Gwen, it's one of the boys. I just don't want to embarrass them. So we'll just say it's Gwen.)

I have tried everything to convince Gwen to go to the toilet. I reasoned with her. I got mad. I ignored the issue to let it run its course. I even stooped so low *(don't tell Alfie!)* as to set up a gold-star system next to the toilet. Nothing worked. Gwen just kept dancing and wiggling and peeing her pants.

Until I read Cohen. And then I gave play a shot. And it won hands down. When I notice that Gwen has to pee and is holding it in, at first I say nothing. I don't want to create a dynamic that separates us, to turn it into me versus her. Cohen taught me that Gwen needs me on her team. So, instead, a few moments later, eyes wide, excited, like it's part of the game we are playing, I say, "Okay, while I shuffle the cards, you see if you can race to the bathroom, pull down your pants, have a pee, and get back before I'm done. Ready, GO!" And off she races.

One of our babysitters had a similar solution. She sets her phone to go off every forty-five minutes. The phone beeps, and she and Gwen drop whatever what they are doing and have a dramatic race to the bathroom. Gwen loves the anticipation. *When will the phone beep?* She giggles the whole way there.

This is not simply about avoiding conflict and stress or getting what I want — for Gwen to pee on potty. These are perks of Playful Parenting, for sure, but the real goal is to allow her to process her feelings. We are connecting and helping Gwen along. Why does she hold it in? I don't know. Maybe she likes having something that she gets to control. Maybe in tensing the muscles in her pelvis, she is building core strength, much as we yogis do in *mula bandha*. Maybe she just likes the sensation. It's kind of stimulating and intense. Try it, and you'll see.

Either way, rather than shaming her or scolding her or detaching from her, which would certainly not help, we connect, and she works through the issue feeling supported and held.

Something as simple as laughter over a silly joke can release all the tension in the house and make everyone feel better. When Gwen chooses to unleash a nice big pee *again* in her pants, I engage her playfully and without annoyance. Or I get annoyed and make a game of my annoyance. Dramatically playing it up with hands on hips, a smile, and a tickle. Then we are a team. We are connected. We are on the same side. And she feels supported and cared for.

I saw my friends Erica and Phil use this stuff recently. Erica and Phil each work three days a week and alternate watching their kids. This was Erica's day with the kids, and it was a long one. She came over to our house at 4:00 PM.

Phil was still at work and showed up an hour later. He wanted to change out of his business suit and Erica had forgotten his shorts. Phil was clearly disappointed and annoyed. Erica snapped, "I remembered to bring the kids' sunscreen, bathing suits, and the diaper bag! That should be enough!"

I loaned him shorts, but Erica and Phil were both pissed at and tense with each other. No one was right, wrong, or at fault. How to move through it? Gwen and I would probably have been sullen for half a day and then talked about it before moving on. A fine solution. But, Phil, a devoted Cohen admirer, grabbed the Super Soaker and drenched Erica. She, in turn, snatched the garden hose and chased him. Soon they were wrestling and roaring with laughter, drenched and reconnected. I thought they were going to have terrific sex right there on the lawn.

I, too, called on Cohen this very morning. Gwen had made a delicious rice cereal for the boys' breakfast. She simmers white basmati rice with milk and cinnamon and raisins and a touch of maple syrup. The boys used to love this, but lately it has gone out of fashion. Ordinarily I listen to that and trust that their bodies know best. Maybe they've had too much of it and need a change. But for today, it is here, and I don't have time to make something else. Starting tomorrow we can take it out of the breakfast rotation for a while. But today, I need them to want it. And they are about to start screaming.

Ever since we toured Connecticut's Thimble Islands, where Captain Kidd hid some of his treasure, the boys have been obsessed with pirates. So I add a cut-up fig and a few dried cranberries and apricots and tell the boys, "Arrg, avast, look yonder!" They look up, wide-eyed, eyes sparkling. "There be pirate treasure in this bowl."

"What does each thing represent?" Noah asks.

I tell him, "The cranberries are rubies, the apricots are gold, and the fig is a treasure chest!" They dig in, eager and giggling.

There are times when I can't do this, if, say, the night before I have had too little sleep or too much beer (basically anything more than one beer). Or, maybe, if I have woken up at 4:00 in the morning to edit this manuscript, so that by 6:30, when the boys wake up, I am ready for a nap. In those cases it's tough to be playful; in those cases it's tough just to answer yes-no questions.

But when I can find the creativity and the energy, this stuff is wizardry. When Benji doesn't want to get into the tub, we become grizzlies and go swimming in the lake. And after Benji spends all morning at a friend's house petting a cat dangerously close to the cat's anus but refuses to wash his hands, I say, "Benji, do you want to try the hand-washing machine?" I place the cloth on my open hands, make a machine sound, and open and close them like a jaw. Benji giggles and puts his hands in the machine for a wash. Score another one for zany Larry Cohen.

Playful Parenting definitely makes life easier, less tense, and more fun. But it's more than that. It helps kids move through the wave of a feeling, rather than having the feeling get blocked or cut off partway. And it helps them connect, feel powerful, and build confidence.

The results of all this are impressive and really delightful. When Noah comes into my room kicking, I ask myself what's really going on for him. And when I engage him with play, he can allow his feelings to be expressed and find resolution and completion. As Cohen points out, "Shared suffering helps us release it."

This stuff is so great and has been so impressively successful that I'm tempted to use all this with Gwen. Next time she's underslept and makes a humphy comment, I'll give her a playful tickle. Next time she's overwhelmed by the laundry, the kids howling, and the mess in the house, I'll just act goofy, like Frankenstein, and pretend to chase her.

What do you think? Great idea? Or a potential crime of passion in the works?

I'll let you know how it goes.

Chapter 31

Kohn Meet Cohen

People just want to be close,
no matter what crazy stupid ways they might show it.

— Larry Cohen, *Playful Parenting*

*T*his morning Benji and Noah are playing in the family room. Noah has made a game of sorting playing cards into categories, and Benji is playing with his farm animals. Soon Benji wants Noah's attention and is getting frustrated. Feeling he has no other options, he hits Noah pretty hard on the head. The classic caveman/two-year-old's approach to courting.

Noah, of course, gets angry. He does not receive Benji's wallop as, "Stop ignoring me; I want to play with you." So he yells at Benji, "Don't hit me!" Benji is happy simply to be in relationship. He says, "Okay," and kicks Noah.

Three more of my hairs just went gray. These days, the boys' fighting is my number one source of stress. *Mental note: Call Dad and Mom later to apologize for the million times that Larry and I wrestled, sparred, and fought. And for the time I hit Larry with an oar. And for the time I bit him and he had to get a tetanus shot.*

I jump off the toilet, pants at my ankles, and rush in before Noah sends Benji flying.

I say, "Benji, we don't hit or kick."

Not bad. Certainly better than, "Benji, you are bad!"

But then I remember Alfie and Larry, and I ask myself, "What is happening here?" I attune. I get conscious. Benji wants Noah's attention. That's pretty much the only reason he'd ever hit him. Noah is Benji's idol. If Benji had his druthers, he'd be interacting with Noah at all times, pausing only for meals and using the potty.

So I say, "Benji, we don't hit or kick. In this family, we kiss and tickle." Benji smiles and says, "Then I will tickle him!" and rushes over and tickles Noah's scalp. Noah laughs and now they are both giggling and wrestling. Benji is elated. He has exactly what he wanted — a connection with Noah.

Instead of focusing on Benji's behavior and punishing him, I followed the Kohn/Cohen brothers' advice and looked deeper at the problem. Instead of doing things *to* Benji, I worked *with* him. Playfully. And it worked better for everyone. Thanks to Alfie and Larry, I got to make a real difference for both my boys.

Then I head back to the bathroom.

Chapter 32

How to Talk So Kids Will Listen and Listen So Kids Will Talk

I ask a lot of questions. I can't help it. I'd have done very well as an agent during the Spanish Inquisition. I'd have risen in the ranks effortlessly. Except for the violence. I have no stomach for violence.

Or maybe I am an interrogator simply because Gwen is Canadian and my kids are, well, kids. Ask a fellow Jew in New Jersey how he or she feels, and you'll get, "Oh, well, my head hurts — a migraine, I think. And my in-laws are visiting and, from me to you to Gawd, they are killing me. Killing me, I tell you. And of course my irritable bowel syndrome is acting up. Thankfully, no blood this time, but a lot of mucus. How are you?"

But Gwen is Canadian, so when I ask her how her day has been, all I get is, "Pretty good, eh? And you?"

I'm thankful for the *eh*. Without it I'd lose 20 percent of the answer.

My kids are equally taciturn. When I ask them about their day, they say absolutely nothing. This leaves me wanting and triggers a fruitless interrogation. So I was very happy to discover Adele Faber and Elaine Mazlish's genius book, *How to Talk So Kids Will Listen & Listen So Kids Will Talk*.

Adele Faber's book begins with a bit of history. Which is awesome. I love discovering the human side of my heroes. Finding out that they, too, struggle makes me feel like less of a complete jackass. So I was happy to discover that the story of Adele and Elaine begins in a parenting class. They were taking a class run by a young psychologist, Dr. Haim Ginott, who would later become the best-selling author of *Between Parent and Child*.

Ginott's class became the foundation for *How to Talk*. In fact, Dr. Ginott popularized many of the holistic alternative parenting memes that we see today in Attachment Parenting workshops, nonviolent communication trainings, and Celestial Seasonings tea boxes.

Ginott taught:

- Do not deny or ignore a child's feelings.
- Treat behavior, never the child, as unacceptable.
- Don't make it personal. "I see an unmade bed" rather than "You didn't make your bed!"
- Use mantras; for example, "Food is not for throwing."
- Let children do for themselves what they can. Nobody likes to be overly dependent.
- Let children choose (within safe limits). "Would you like your yellow duck or your blue ship in the tub with you?"
- Don't use *never* or *always*, as in: "You never clean up." Instead, refer to a specific event.
- Don't use words or phrases that you don't want to hear from your child.

Faber and Mazlish's first book was actually a memoir of their experiences applying what they had learned in Ginott's classes. In this book, they never preached or even tried to teach anything. They figured that parents would read their story and be inspired to apply it in their own parenting. Rather than saying, "Parent this way," they modeled it in their memoir. Which is pretty cool and a great example of Adele and Elaine walking their talk.

But parents loved the memoir and wanted more. They begged Faber and Mazlish for a how-to manual with lessons and drills, and thus was born *How to Talk So Kids Will Listen & Listen So Kids Will Talk.*

So, what's all the hype? Do their approaches really work? They do. And they are magic.

Here's Faber and Mazlish's basic approach:

1. *When your kids speak, listen with full attention.*
2. *Rather than responding with questions and advice, acknowledge your child's feelings with, "Oh...mmm...I see."*
3. *Give your child's feeling a name.* Acknowledge her experience. For example, say, "That sounds frustrating."
4. *(optional) You can even authentically acknowledge their feelings with fantasy:* "I *wish* I could make the pizza be ready right now!" I think Playful Parenting would work very well here. I can see a wooden spoon as wand, some magic words, and lots of giggling and bonding.

Of course, that last step could also seem mocking or patronizing, so I might need to practice being attuned. Some kids, I suspect, really just like silence and cuddles when they feel hurt, and others like their feelings to be named. If I pay attention, with time and practice, I know I will learn to see clearly.

When a child comes to us and says that someone took his toy or that he is tired, we can deny the feeling by saying, "Well, you didn't put it away," or "No, that's impossible, you just napped," but this confuses the child. He may feel dismissed and ignored, or, worse, belittled and patronized.

But if we respond with supportive nods and sounds or simply

affirming and naming their feelings, "Mmm, someone took your toy," and "You're tired," kids feel supported and validated. They feel safe having feelings, and they learn to trust their feelings. They feel empowered to find solutions or simply to move on. And they see they are not alone in their struggles. Instead of meltdowns, this approach triggers a sigh and steps toward resolution.

I find this same phenomenon in meditation. When I stop trying to control and change the way I feel and, instead, simply observe or even name it, my feelings flow more easily, my body relaxes, and I feel a new energy and vitality.

I have seen this work time and again with my boys. The only difficulty is in remembering to use it. I want to jump right into solving a problem or pointing out someone's error. I have to remember to hold myself back and follow the formula.

Take last week.

Noah was drawing a birthday card for his cousin, Natalia, when Benji bumped his arm, giving the N in *Natalia* a tail. Noah was distraught and furious. I wanted to say, "Benji didn't mean it," or "Here's an eraser," or even, "It's just a card." But saying any of that would throw fresh fuel on the fire. Luckily, I remembered *How to Talk So Kids Will Listen & Listen So Kids Will Talk*, so I said to Noah, "Mmm. Benji bumped you?"

"Yes!"

"That sounds frustrating."

"Yes, it is! He ruined my picture!"

"Oh. *(earnest, not patronizing)* It's ruined?"

"Yes! *(calming down)* Well, no, actually, I can probably erase the mistake."

Done. Magic. Noah moves on. Thank you, Adele Faber and Elaine Mazlish.

By the way, probably the single most important thing I've incorporated from their genius book is simply "Don't ask too many questions," especially at greetings.

I don't want to seem melodramatic when I say this has changed my life. When I get home from work, I am overflowing with questions for Gwen and the boys. How was school? Any problems? What did you learn in knitting class? Is everyone safe and happy? Did you like the lunch I packed?

But team *How to Talk* has taught me to simply say, "So glad to see you." This takes every ounce of discipline I can muster. I am chomping at the bit to unleash a sortie of interrogations.

When I slip up or can't restrain myself and I greet Gwen and the boys with a barrage of questions, they get overwhelmed and shut down. They run from me or get angry. But when I can hold back and I greet the boys with, "So glad so see you," they glow. We sit together and read or run around and chase each other or sing "Supercalifragilisticexpialidocious." We connect.

I can only wait so long, so eventually I sneak in the questions, but I'm working on postponing as long as possible, ideally until, in passing, they wind up telling me of their own accord about their day.

If this was all Faber and Mazlish ever gave us, that would have been enough. Dayenu. But there's more! Next they tackle discipline.

When children behave in a way that is inappropriate, Faber and Mazlish recommend:

1. *Describe what you see.* "The breakfast dishes are still on the table."

2. *Give information.* It's less personal and seems less like an attack, so it's easier to take in. Plus, information allows children (and adults!) to figure out for themselves what needs to be done. "The table won't be clear when it's time for lunch."

3. *The shorter the reminder, the better.* Maybe even just one word. Rather than, "You forgot, *AGAIN*, to take off

your muddy shoes and leave them on the mat! You are tracking mud all over!" you can simply say, "Shoes." You've probably been through this discussion many times, and your kids will know exactly what you mean. And they will respond. They will feel less lectured and they will probably stop, take their shoes off, and place them on the mat. If instead, you go into a rant, they will certainly feel worse and less empowered, and strangely, they probably won't take off the shoes and put them on the mat.

Short words or phrases are so much less preachy, and let's face it, our kids already know what we are going to say. This is probably just as true for adults. I'd say Gwen and I have a total of, like, three fights and we just play them out in different ways. How nice if we could just note the fight with a word, "Shoes," and skip the whole business.

4. *Talk about your own feelings, not about the child's character or personality*. This keeps out the judgment and guilt. "I don't like eating at a dirty, crowded table."

5. *(optional) Write a note or speak from the object's point of view*. "Please clean me so I'm ready for lunch. Thanks! — Your Table." Again, I think, Larry Cohen would find this last step wonderfully playful!

This approach to discipline allows us to teach our kids without judging or blaming them. As Faber says, "Sometimes it takes no more than a few words, a look, or a tone of voice to tell you that you're either 'slow or stupid,' 'a pest,' or a basically likable and capable person. How your parents think of you can often be communicated in seconds. When you multiply those seconds by the hours of daily contact between parents and children, you begin to realize how powerfully young people can be influenced by the way their parents view them."

All this stuff is amazing. Unbelievable. Try it. You'll be shocked.

And, again, there's more! After *How to Talk* Faber and Mazlish wrote the follow-up book, *Siblings without Rivalry,* which is basically the same but for more than one kid.

Today Gwen used it with the boys. They were all on our bed reading stories. Gwen was in the middle, between the two boys. This is very sweet, and when I come home to this, I want to hang my hat on a hook, click my heels together, and wink to the camera.

But today it was a powder keg. Noah was home from school with a cold. This distracted Benji from his routine, and he hadn't napped. Gwen was reading *Make Way for Ducklings.* Noah has all the words memorized and is "reading" along. Benji doesn't want Noah to do this, and Noah doesn't want to stop. Soon everyone will be screaming, crying, and tearing at their hair.

But Gwen saves the day. She simply acknowledges each boy's feelings. And that dissipates it. Instead of controlling things, she says, "Noah wants to say the words. And Benji does not want him to. *(pause)* What can we do about this?"

No one had a solution, but they didn't even need one. Everyone felt heard. And now they were reconnected. And that was enough. They talked for a moment, everyone felt better, and Gwen kept reading.

This is all very magical for the kids, but what about for your husband or wife? I think it works just as well. In all our relationships and interactions, we just want to be seen and heard and acknowledged. We want to be connected. If Gwen and I are fighting and I am making a point and Gwen does not respond, I will say it over and over until she nods or disagrees. She hates this. But, until she acknowledges me, I feel like a ship lost at sea.

So Faber and Mazlish's formula is genius, even with adults. Though, perhaps, we need to use it a bit more subtly.

My favorite author, A. J. Jacobs, wrote a hilarious piece about this (in *My Life as an Experiment*). Impressed with the success of *How to Talk*'s approach on his five-year-old, he tried it out on his wife, Julie, when she was angry that he'd lent out a DVD to their nanny without asking.

JULIE: "You lent it to Michelle without asking me?"

A.J: "I lent it to Michelle." *(Repeating.)* "I'm sorry."

JULIE: "I was going to watch it tonight."

A.J.: "You were going to watch it tonight? Tonight?"

JULIE: "I'd planned this out for a couple of days."

A.J.: "Mmm."

JULIE: "This is the second time you've done this."

A.J.: "I can see how that would be really annoying."

She paused.

JULIE: "Do *not* talk to me like you talk to the boys."

Damn. She figured it out? Was I too obvious?

A.J.: "Don't talk to you like I talk to the boys?" I asked.

JULIE: "The tone. It's the tone you use with Jasper."

A.J.: "That must be frustrating."

JULIE: "Stop it!"

Chapter 33

Poop

Knock, knock.
Who's there?
Iatemyp.
Iatemyp who?
Oh! You ate your poo?!

— Noah's favorite knock-knock joke

For much of your life, you don't deal with other people's pee and poop. Until you become a parent. Then, you have a pee and poop PhD. You're knee-deep.

One day last year I was reading while Benji was playing with his farm animals. Suddenly, he gets up, toddles off to his little Baby-Björn potty, pulls down his pants, and sits for a poop. I almost cried. I ran to tell Gwen. But first I squinted my face and pressed my fingers into my temples to commit the scene to memory. This way I can always come back to it.

I don't feel the same way when anyone else, say, Gwen or my brother, goes to the bathroom. Big toilets and adult poop are simply not as cute. Nature has truly succeeded here in guaranteeing that we care for our young — even their poop is adorable. A good thing, since we deal with it quite a lot.

Parents become fascinated by poop. They talk about it at dinner. Even Al Bundy–like men who wince at the idea of changing a diaper are surprised to find infant poop delightful.

This isn't so odd, considering that the rest of the animal kingdom treats poop with tremendous respect. Many parents in the animal kingdom identify their progeny by their poop smell. Some go so far as to sneak a nibble here and there to cement the scent in their mind. I haven't taken it quite that far, though I think Gwen is concerned.

Before I was a dad, I attended a family gathering of our friends Hillary and Clive. Hillary and Clive's daughter, Edna, was learning to use a potty. She was walking around naked, and I remember she let one loose on the rug right in the middle of the room. Hillary shouts, "Poop!" and Clive scoops up little Edna and rushes her to the potty while Clive's brother, whose house (and rug) it is, simply grabs a napkin and scoops up the poop like after a puppy on the lawn. I don't even think there's much of a scrub. At the time, before I had my own kids, I would have expected white vinegar, bleach, and maybe calling in for air support to fire-bomb the whole sector.

Poop becomes a part of your psyche. Just this morning, as I woke up, Gwen cuddled up next to me and whispered, "I had a dream that I was sitting on the monkey bars at the playground. A girl, maybe Noah's friend Aruni, climbed onto my lap."

"That's sweet," I whispered.

"Yes," she continued, "but then suddenly she has no pants on and she pooped on me. It got all over my new Ibex yoga pants. You know the black merino wool pair. *(shaking her head)* The dream felt so real."

Before my parenting training, I would either have nodded and moved on or offered an inspiring, "Good thing it wasn't true." But now that I've read *How to Talk So Kids Will Listen & Listen So Kids Will Talk*, I know to validate Gwen's feelings and say, "Mmm...On your Ibex pants?...That sounds upsetting."

"Yes," she confirmed, "it was."

Feeling heard and validated, she smiled, stretched, and got up. She went straight to her pants drawer and smiled again at her beloved yoga pants, poop-free and intact.

Chapter 34

Divorce

There are only two ways to live your life.
One is as though nothing is a miracle.
The other is as though everything is a miracle.

— Albert Einstein

*P*arenting kinda sucks.

And it's also the best thing ever. Often at exactly the same time.

This morning, for example, I was tired and in no mood for *usual.* That's what Noah and I call our morning ritual of playing a game or drawing a picture together on the couch after he wakes up. I was even less in the mood for Gwen to be underslept and grumpy and for Benji to be three years old and in tears if I sliced his French toast in the wrong direction. Which I did. So this morning sucked.

And it was also miraculous. Gwen was in the bathroom with Noah, brushing his hair. I was standing in the kitchen checking email on my iPhone while Benji finished his breakfast at the kitchen table. I watched as he ate. He's at the stage of being exactly the size of a small Ewok. He even moves like one and he has an Ewok's focus and attention. He was totally absorbed in the work of eating his breakfast. First his French toast. Then, with a *don't mind if I do* glance, he moved his French toast plate out of the way and swapped in his bowl of oatmeal.

Benji now attends a nursery program two mornings a week. Last week, his teacher taught him to lean over his oatmeal bowl during snack so that he'll drip into the bowl and not onto his sweater. So this morning he sits up a bit straighter to get some height and bends over the bowl to avoid spilling. The way he leans forward with his tiny body, so intentional, jutting his neck out to drip into the bowl, is so cute I am swooning. Sometimes the love is almost too much to hold. For a split second, my knees go weak; I'm a preteen girl at a Justin Bieber concert.

One minute I am stressed and miserable. The next, I sigh, my body softens, and I could not be happier. Literally. The highs are so high, they completely dissolve the lows.

And what's the alternative, anyway? What did I do that was so great when I actually had time? Would I rather be sitting on the couch watching a movie? Going to a yoga class? Sleeping in? No. Of course not. Okay, yes. Yes, I would.

But not really. As *New York* magazine concluded in their famous 2010 article "All Joy and No Fun," day to day, parents are less happy and more stressed, but in the long run they feel a deep sense of purpose and are more satisfied.

So having kids exposes you to transcendent moments of love, connection, and happiness, but day to day, everyone is stressed, no one is sleeping, and there hasn't been sex in weeks or even months. This is why it is *not* a good time to make big life decisions.

I have a little rule for myself. Before I ram the car in front of me for driving below the speed limit, I ask myself, "Have I slept less than seven consecutive hours, eaten six brownies, or had a fight with Gwen?" If the answer to any of these questions is yes, then I give the driver a second chance before he meets the front end of my Corolla.

The same must be true for our partners.

We must advocate for our needs but also give them time and space. And we must accept a certain amount of chaos and discord.

Bottom line, I don't think couples with small children should be allowed to divorce. With no time to connect, lacking sleep, and always feeling overwhelmed, parents of very small children, it seems to me, are not of sound mind to make such a life-changing decision. Unless they are. Sometimes divorce, I suppose, is the only option. Obviously if there is abuse. Or if partners realize that they are truly incompatible.

But otherwise, the person you married will likely return in a few years when the kids are older, and a divorce would screw all that up.

After Gwen gave birth, she changed from Anne of Green Gables to Beowolf. (I think it's been long enough, now, that I can joke about this. Right, honey? Honey?) And I don't really blame her; years of not sleeping and putting your own needs third will do that to a person.

But then, like the Hulk returning to David Banner, slowly, over time, she returned. One morning she woke up, blinked a few times, and said, "Whoa, where have I been?" And that was it; my Gwen was back. God forbid we had divorced; I'd have missed out on a lifetime of loving her.

Chapter 35

Germophobia

My sister, Julie, is a bit of a germophobe. No more than I was, but she's not a parent, so she hasn't spent countless hours squatting in public restroom stalls begging her toddler not to lick the wall. Having small children breaks you of any germ fears. There is no other choice.

This past weekend Julie drove with my boys and me to New Jersey to visit our folks. We stop off the highway at a chain restaurant for lunch, and before we get back in the car, Julie takes the boys to the bathroom for one last pee before hitting the road.

About to wash his hands, Noah asks Aunt Julie if his new ring from the Tooth Fairy is waterproof. Julie isn't sure, so to be safe, Noah takes it off and sets it on a folded paper towel.

Sensible enough. But Julie accidentally overturns the paper towel.

No one sees where the ring goes, though they hear a soft *ping* as it lands somewhere.

They get down and look around. Now, keep in mind that, as mentioned, Julie is not accustomed to kneeling in public restrooms.

She has never had to hold back a scream as she watches Benjamin squeeze his tiny body behind the toilet tank. She has never had to stand in puddles of unidentified liquid as she wipes tiny tushies. She has never had to fish out a fallen potty ring from very unclean toilet water.

So kneeling on the tile bathroom floor at O'Mally's already demonstrates the great love that Aunt Julie has for her nephews.

Still, she can't see any sign of the ring. Impossible. It's not on the counter. It's not on the floor. A woman in one of the stalls catches on to the urgency of their quest and loans Julie a flashlight from her purse. Clearly a mom.

I look in the hallway, in case the ring has rolled out, and eventually we clear the women's bathroom so I can join in on the search.

Then it dawns on Julie. There is only one other possibility. The ring must have bounced off the sink counter and into the trash barrel. This is a big trash bin. No need to empty this thing more than once a day; it contains a hearty abundance of used paper towels, snotty tissues, bloody pads, soiled wipes, and lumpy chewing gum.

But Julie earns her aunt badge that day as she rolls up her sleeves and digs in. Up to her shoulder.

Still no ring.

By now the management has been alerted. A man in a headset fires off commands to Lost and Found, our waitress, and someone named Edna for backup.

Edna comes to the bathroom and carries the trash barrel to the back of the kitchen to search through it. Meanwhile, Julie dumps her purse in case that's where the ring is hiding.

Five minutes later Edna emerges from the kitchen, and she is holding…the ring.

I cheer. Noah is thrilled. Julie jumps into the air.

And then thoroughly washes her hand, arm, and shoulder.

Chapter 36

Simplicity Parenting

Simplify, simplify, simplify.

— Henry David Thoreau

I love this Thoreau quote. Though, really, let's face it, it might
have been said a bit more simply. One *simplify* certainly could
have done the trick.

Of this, author Kim John Payne should take note. He has written a lovely book about simplifying the lives of our children and our
families. But the book is in, like, a 9-point font. How can you publish
a book on simplicity and use a 9-point font? Make it one large word
per page. Maybe with an illustrative photo or cartoon. Now, that
would be simple. Really, he needed only seven pages. Just the words
do less, one letter per page.

I had been putting this book off, waiting for the illustrated edi-
tion. But, when I finally do dig in, Payne is no disappointment.

We want our kids to be successful, of course. But the way to help
them be successful, says Payne, is not what you might think. It is
not to sign them up for Mandarin lessons at age five. It is not to start
them early on SAT prep or play them Bach through in-utero speak-
ers. It is to give them space. To channel *Little House on the Prairie*.
To pretend for a few years that you are Amish. Unplug the TV. Just

give 'em a corncob and let them invent games and use it alternately as a doll, a magic wand, and a bulldozer. Heck, if they get a bit peckish before dinner, they can even have a nibble.

Payne says that right from the cradle we overwhelm kids with too much structure and scheduled activity. "There is an undeclared war on childhood," says Payne. The solution? More time mucking around the creek. More time wrestling with a difficult homework question before checking the Internet. More time spent quietly in the den. These dull moments, says Payne, are when inspiration hits. And they teach us the patience and fortitude necessary to deal with difficult issues in adulthood.

By the way, when I eventually show this chapter to Payne he is a terrific sport and receives my playful *Little House on the Prairie* jabs with humor. Still, he points out that Simplicity Parenting is not at all a return to the past. On the contrary, it prepares children for the future.

He tells me, "The average stay in a job in the United States is now 2.7 years, and more and more jobs are either contract, part-time, or self-created. If our children are to succeed in this kind of world, then we need to allow them the time and space to cultivate creativity, innovation, and adaptability inwardly."

Payne writes more about this in his book:

When we really look at what happens for a kid when they slow down, tune in to themselves, take space and get busy in serious play, we can see that what they are learning is how to create a kind of inner structure that will serve them (and us) well in the world ahead.... The great news is that we don't have to do that much to introduce our kids to the benefits of their own intelligence and freedom. Just relax a little bit. Give them just a bit more space than you think you can.

This makes sense to me, in many ways. For example, when Noah comes home from school with tear streaks on his eyeglasses, I want to grill him, find out what the problem is, call his teacher, and work it out. Make it better for him. I want perfect harmony in Noah's life.

But when I ask about the tears, Noah resists me. He wants to work it out on his own or let it run its course. And I can see now that that is exactly what he needs. He needs me to give him a bit more space than I am comfortable with. Space to sit with it. Space to build his emotional muscles. Space to figure it out on his own.

If he asked for my help or if there were signs of bullying or inappropriate behavior, I'd jump right in, of course. But, otherwise, forcing my way in would only meet my needs and soothe my anxiety, not his.

Within this space, Noah can develop his own communication skills, fortitude, and inner strength. I would do him no service by micromanaging his every conflict. This would steal from him the opportunity to exercise his own muscles. It would teach him that his challenges make me worried, that I don't trust he can handle them.

Payne recommends that we bring this spaciousness to all levels of our lives. He recommends that we simplify our

- *Environment:* decluttering all the stuff that fills the shelves, chests, and toy bins at home
- *Rhythm:* increasing predictability and allowing time for connection and calm
- *Schedule*: allowing quiet, unstructured time
- *Kids' experience of the adult world:* reducing the influence of adult concerns, media, and consumerism on children

Payne finds that taking these steps helps children feel calmer and happier, more comfortable socially, and more able to focus. This simplicity, Payne notes, can sometimes take a child with ADHD or Asperger's and put them back into alignment.

Moreover, Payne finds that parents on the plan develop a clearer picture of what they value as parents, are more united in their parenting, and have more time and energy for connection, relaxation, and fun.

That makes pretty good sense. I know that the quieter my environment, the easier it is for me to feel and hear my own parenting instincts and intuition. And I can use a dose of Payne's medicine. Right now, our life feels just bananas.

I'm wondering where to start, so I've been trolling parenting blogs for reviews of Payne's book, and I see that most families focus on the first level of simplification, the environment.

This step involves, basically, clearing out toys from the family room. Payne says, "As you decrease the quantity of your child's toys and clutter, you increase their attention and their capacity for deep play....A smaller, more manageable quantity of toys invites deeper play and engagement. An avalanche of toys invites emotional disconnect and overwhelm."

Payne says that when kids are overwhelmed, they freak out. And he provides some very compelling anecdotes, one, for example, about two brothers who freak out every time they enter the playroom. But after the clutter is cleared, they get along and play blissfully.

Word of warning: We are not talking here about putting a few toys in the basement. This is not about tidying the den. No. We are talking about reducing clutter by a magnitude of 90 percent. We are talking about a return to Depression-era, post–stock market crash, Herbert Hoover America.

Payne recommends retaining only the three toys your children use most. And they should be toys that foster imagination. Payne favors toys that are not "fixed," that do only one thing. If you push a button and only one thing can happen, the toy is fixed. This includes Furby, LOL Elmo, Barbie, and any Hannah Montana doll. These allow children to recount the TV show or commercial but do not invite imagination. They celebrate Hollywood, not our children.

The opposite is a toy that a child can pour their imagination into, such as a pile of blocks that can be transformed into anything of which a child dreams. Payne favors simple toys made of natural materials. These are tactually stimulating and give a child's imagination free rein to frolic. They invite exploration.

Payne tells us to start by removing broken toys, toys your child has outgrown or not yet grown into, overly complex toys such as a rocket that shoots a missile and blinks lights and turns into a soldier, high-stimulation toys with lots of sound and lights, toys that claim to give a developmental edge, and multiples. Just because Billy loves his stuffed bunny does not mean we should buy him fifteen more. In fact, that would dilute the sacredness of little Wey Wey bunny.

I feel Payne's pain, and I appreciate his prognosis. I think this is genius and will have amazing benefits.

For you.

But I am from New Jersey. If you've seen *Jersey Shore*, you know that I have already done a pretty good job of simplifying. It all started when I gave up hair gel. From there everything went fairly easily. I gave away my television. We have a lot of toys, but none of them buzz, beep, or speak. Noah and Benji's toys only move when they push them. We have lots of wood in the den. We even paid $104 for a wooden marble run when we could have gotten the plastic version for $28. That's all I can do for now. I'm not ready to channel the Great Depression into our den.

Actually, the night I read Payne's chapter, Gwen and I discuss it and do plan, at least, to start culling toys the following day.

But that evening, we get a call from my sister crying, saying that my dad has been diagnosed with stage IV lung and bone cancer. We knew he had been having some pain, was unaccountably sleepy, and had gone to the hospital for a CAT scan, but we had no idea the results would be so grim. In shock, we prepare to head down to New Jersey.

Lying in bed at night, I think about what to tell the boys, especially Noah, who is seven and old enough to understand. He already knows that Grandpa Manny is sick and went to the hospital for a test.

We don't know how long my dad has. Could be years. My gut tells me much, much less. We decide to follow Payne's lead: *Simplify kids' experience of the adult world — reduce the influence of adult concerns on children.*

We won't use adult words. We will allow Noah to experience my dad directly without intellectualizing. He will understand on a much deeper level. And without all the anxiety and fear that words like *cancer* evoke, even in a seven-year-old.

The following day, we drive to New Jersey. In the backseat, the boys make cards for my dad. "We Love You, Grandpa Manny."

When we arrive, my dad is in a large electric hospital bed in the family room. Noah and Benji run in, all smiles, and reach up on tiptoes to greet my dad with a kiss on the cheek. They give him the cards and pictures they drew. And then, as usual, they run off to play with their favorite toys from the closet in the playroom.

At lunch, they chat with my dad, asking each other the usual questions. My dad asks, "How's school?" Noah answers and asks my dad if he knows how many countries are in Africa. Benji just watches, taking it all in. They can see that my dad has trouble keeping his head up. They see that his eyes look heavy.

When my dad has to use the bathroom, I walk him slowly to the toilet and steady him while he pees. Noah and Benji watch. Deep down they understand what is happening but they never look worried. They see reality as it is, simple and direct, without labels and anxiety.

When my dad dies, I don't think it will trigger fears or anxieties for Noah or Benji. Grappling with the intellectual concept of cancer, especially at their age, might cause them anxiety. They might ask, "Will it kill my dad, too?"

But the direct experience of Grandpa Manny, of seeing him, will not trigger these fears. They see him simply as he is. They see reality as it is. They will not extrapolate his condition onto me. Concepts cause anxiety. Direct experience of reality does not.

So far Gwen and I have not sorted the toys in the house. But I am forever grateful to Kim John Payne for sharing his wisdom exactly when my family needed it most.

Chapter 37

Sex

Years ago, toward the end of a month-long program at Kripalu, I found myself sitting in the hot tub next to a very famous yogi. I knew he had recently left the order of monks and was in a relationship, and I wondered how often an ex-monk has sex.

So I asked him, "How often do you have sex?"

Ever equanimous, he equivocated, "There's no certain prescription. But ideally, for me, sex should not be stress management or a way to smooth over a fight. My partner and I have sex when we feel a bubbling up of love for each other and the urge to express that love physically."

Very nice. Beautiful answer. But I want a number.

I push him, "So this bubbling up of love happens, what, a few times a day, monthly, only on solstice?"

"Okay, okay," he relents, "about once a month."

At the time, at age twenty-five, that sounded awfully slim to me. But now, at age forty, as father to two young children, from what

I hear from fellow parents, once a month, if you average it all out, seems a lot less out-there.

Moral of the story?

Once you have kids, your sex life gets a lot more yogic.

Chapter 38

Meditation

Sometimes on a Saturday afternoon, after the family has been together all day, I like to meditate. Correction. Sometimes on a Saturday afternoon, after the family has been together all day, I *need* to meditate.

But it's difficult for me to meditate in my house if everyone is home. Not because of the noise. I have no problem with that. Hearing the boys playing in the background is Krishna Das and bamboo flutes to my ears. And it's also not because the boys don't want me to meditate. Not at all. They love when I meditate. Which is why it's so difficult. Because they like to join me.

Now, don't get me wrong. This is a dream come true. My boys now think meditation is the bee's knees and can't wait to have at it. They even have their own cushions. So I should be ecstatic about this. And I am. Hopefully it will initiate a lifelong love of meditation, spirituality, and holistic health.

But it gets in the way of my own practice. For example, last year Noah invented an aura-cleansing technique that he employed while I meditated. He'd have made a fine Peruvian shaman. He'd gather several colors of silk scarves, a whistle, and two rhythm sticks, and as I meditated he'd circle me waving the scarves, banging the sticks, chanting, and every now and then blowing a shrill screech on the whistle. It definitely cleansed my aura. Though by the end of each sit, I was a nervous wreck.

This year, he's into sitting. And Benji imitates him. So when they catch me meditating, they each get out their cushions. We settle in. We sit quietly.

Noah closes his eyes and peeks at me every few seconds. Benji closes his eyes, which is a real effort when you are three years old. His whole face works in unison, scrunching to keep his eyes closed. After a minute or two, Noah is done and starts an *om*. Benji joins in. As do I. At a total of two minutes, it is a much shorter meditation than I had in mind, but the full-family *om* makes Gwen swoon, and I can see from the adoring look on her face that there just might be sex tonight.

Chapter 39

Ayurveda

When Benji was an infant, he had an angry skin rash on his hands and face. Noah, on the other hand, has never had a skin rash but gets congested easily.

Which makes perfect sense. At least according to the traditional medical system of India, called Ayurveda.

Ayurveda, often called the sister science of yoga, is a system of medicine that has been practiced in India for thousands of years. According to Ayurveda, every person is a blend of three proclivities, or *doshas,* described as ether/air *(vata)*, fire *(pitta)*, and water/earth *(kapha)*. While each person is blend of these energies, usually one predominates.

Ayurveda offers a lot of help with understanding ourselves, our partners, and our kids. I studied Ayurveda in the 1990s, but it's been a while, so Gwen and I take the following survey, designed especially for parents, to confirm our constitutions.

1. When I am cooking breakfast while the kids are asking me questions and the dog is running through the kitchen, I become _____.

      A. scattered and anxious

      B. focused and angry

      C. deer in the headlights

2.   When I'm hungry at a restaurant and the kids are melting down, I primarily get _____.

      A. scattered and anxious

      B. angry

      C. stuck and depressed

3.   When the kids won't bathe unless I get in too, I dread the feeling of being _____.

      A. too cold

      B. too hot

      C. too wet

4.   My biggest parenting struggles involve _____.

      A. worry, fear

      B. impatience, anger

      C. feeling stuck

5.   When I have quickly eaten dinner standing up and it consists of a mismatched smorgasbord of my kids' leftovers, I get _____.

      A. intestinal gas and bloating

      B. heartburn

      C. slow digestion, stagnation

6.   When my kids are sick and wipe their drool and snot on me and I get sick, I experience _____.

      A. worry, feeling fried, constipation

      B. fevers, skin rashes, diarrhea

      C. congestion, feeling blocked up

Mostly As indicates *vata*, mostly Bs *pitta*, and mostly Cs *kapha*. I've got straight As, so *vata dosha*, the energy of air, predominates my constitution. This describes me well. It means that I am on the thin side. It means I get cold easily. I tend to worry. When I get sick or too worried, I can get constipated. It means that sitting in an uncomfortable position reading *Good Night Moon* five times in a row to Benji while he's on his potty gets very tiring and, honestly, a bit dull for me.

That's the downside. But there's an upside, too. There are perks to being an airhead. I am terrifically creative, flexible, and adaptable. As a parent this means I am able to come up with fun games while waiting for an airplane. I can roll with last-minute changes. And I am sensitive and intuitive and can read the boys' moods and needs.

Gwen's survey results, on the other hand, show a fair bit of *kapha* (water/earth) in her constitution, which matches what we know about her. She is earthy. She has a larger frame. *Now, hold on a minute.* Anyone who knows Gwen will understand that I am *not* saying she's a big woman. Gwen is as svelte as I. But if she gave up yoga and ate Big Macs all day, Gwen would gain weight a lot faster than I would. Gwen literally has bigger bones than I do. Put another way, her knuckles are wider than mine. All right, I admit it! When we were shopping for wedding rings, the saleslady suggested I buy a ladies' ring for myself. There it is. I've said it. Now, can we move on?

This also means Gwen is grounded, steady, and reliable. She is steadfast and has endurance. In a *Good Night Moon* reading marathon, she'll win every time.

And Gwen does not worry like I do. She's not worried about whether the tuna has gone bad. She has never asked me to sniff leftovers in the fridge. And she is not obsessed about whether we have black mold (the deadliest kind!) in our walls. I have never seen it, but I am sure it's there.

Gwen is also a bit less creative and flexible. She needs time to adjust to changes. Making up a game for the boys while waiting for a delayed airline flight is stressful for her.

I mentioned that when I get sick or too worried, I can get constipated. What about Gwen? Well, Ayurveda has a lot to say about this, but we'll have to leave it at that. I'm not allowed to discuss Gwen's bowel movements in this book. This was clearly stipulated at the very beginning of the project.

Knowing all this helps us understand each other and helps us parent. It explains why I love to give an impromptu puppet show and why being asked to do so will make Gwen sweat and run from the room.

It explains why she can keep her head straight when packing the car for a winter hike, while I would get scattered and forget somebody's mittens. Every time. Somehow Gwen not only remembers all the mittens but also packs a personalized snack and water bottle for each of us. It also explains why she's the one to carry Benji on her back during the hike. She's just built stronger than I am.

It explains why eating half a bag of chips at night might actually make me feel grounded but leave Gwen feeling glued to the sofa. And why the thought of trekking on an elephant in Thailand puts Gwen in rapture. But for me, though I love the idea of it, and the person I fantasize about being does exactly this sort of thing, in reality, I know that the experience would leave me ungrounded, anxious, and surely flatulent.

Out of balance, the three constitutional types, *vata*, *pitta*, and *kapha*, present with different physical symptoms. Benji's eczema, or any kind of inflamed skin rash, is a sure sign of a *pitta* imbalance. And Noah's mucus congestion is owing to a *kapha* imbalance.

Basically, if someone deals with worry, dryness, and constipation, she's probably *vata*. If she is often angry, too hot, and gets rashes, she's probably *pitta*. And if she is calm, has a bigger build, moves slowly, and often seems stuck, she's probably *kapha*.

The best part of Ayurveda is that by implementing changes to diet, exercise, and routine, I can minimize symptoms and maximize strengths.

The therapies in Ayurveda can be simple lifestyle tweaks (like soaking in some moonlight), complex herbal mixtures, and esoteric recommendations (such as vomit therapy, medical enemas, or a good leeching). I tend to favor the simple remedies. I like to leave the leeching to the pros.

There's a great list of simple Ayurvedic remedies for each constitution in the appendix, along with a more comprehensive Ayurvedic Constitutional Survey.

I attempt to apply all six *vata* therapies from the list. As best a parent can. *Wear soft clothing* I can make happen. Consider it done. *Avoid or cut back on caffeine, wheat, sugar, and processed foods* is trickier. Mostly the sugar part. After a long day, the coconut milk ice cream calls out to me from the freezer. But I'll try. Then there's *Eat at a table, in a relaxed setting*. This one is not gonna happen.

Still, I find these lifestyle changes very powerful. The more I follow them, the more grounded and focused I feel.

Yet, even more powerful, I think, is the insight into Gwen and the boys that the Ayurvedic model provides. I can use the information to help my boys stay balanced and healthy. I can get better insight into Gwen, instead of only interpreting her needs through my own. I can really see why the elephant ride in Thailand is so important to her (*kapha* types thrive on adventure), so I can compromise and make the trip (maybe when the boys are done with college). Hopefully, I can even use some *vata*-balancing therapies to stay grounded along the way. Though this one might require some of those professional touches.

Chapter 40

Never Skip Lunch

Yesterday I spent the night in a hotel in New Haven, Connecticut. It was bliss. And all I really did was get there at 9:00 PM, eat two small bags of chips, drink a can of club soda, flip TV channels, sleep through the night, wake up on my own when my body was ready, go back to sleep, get out of bed, do yoga, eat a very mediocre hotel breakfast, shower, and go to my book talk. This was heaven. Absolute paradise.

And I kept thinking, what if Gwen was here too? We could relax. And cuddle. Maybe even have sex if we could remember how. We might have to call the porter for tips. He could stand over us and give pointers. I'm fairly sure that porters have a lot of sex. Actually, I'm fairly sure that anyone without young children has a lot of sex.

The next day, I get home from my retreat to a total debacle. We start the day at a three-year-old's birthday party. A terrific party, actually. But Gwen and I forget to make sure our two boys eat a proper lunch during the festivities. So when we get home, we set the boys at the kitchen table for a big snack. By now, though, they are beyond hungry and bursting with agitation and emotion. Powder kegs.

Gwen checks our voice mail and finds that our babysitter has canceled. Gwen and I were supposed to have a date. Gwen is devastated.

We let the boys know that our babysitter, whom they adore, is not coming. Explosion. First Noah is screaming. This is too much for little Benji and so, like a domino, he, too, is beside himself. Gwen scoops up Benji. I sit with Noah. Between sobs he eats his tuna and settles down. So does Benji.

After lunch they play happily for twenty minutes. We watch each of them put on a puppet show. Then Gwen and I steal away to hatch a plan. We'll head to a playground and then go out to dinner.

The playground is a lot of fun.

Then dinner. Our biggest mistake of the day. We decide to go to our date restaurant. It'll be fun. They have amazing French fries (and duck gravy for dipping).

We park. We get seated. We order. Noah's mac and cheese arrives. So does Benji's shrimp. Benji sees Noah's noodles and wants them. Noah does not want to give them up. He is a kid and does not say, "I'm sorry, but I don't think I'd like to share that." Instead, he says, "Ahhhhhhhhhh!!!!!!!!!!!"

And of course this knocks over little Benji, who joins in on the chorus with absolute gusto. We are in a fancy restaurant. Noah and Benji are the only children there, and they are screaming at the top of their lungs. People are drinking $9 glasses of Shiraz and nano-brewed beers. I look across the table and Gwen is hiding under her napkin. Literally. As if it's a large sombrero.

By the way, I forgot to mention that Gwen had left her sweater in the car, so as a shawl, draped casually over her shoulders, she is wearing a pair of Noah's sweatpants from the diaper bag. She looks quite elegant in her sweatpants shawl and cloth napkin hat.

So Benji wants the mac and cheese. Noah screams and won't share. I tell him to give Benji some noodles and I'll order more. He acquiesces. I order more. Benji and Noah devour both portions. With a whirl of my arm, like a sailor in a bar, I order another round. "Keep 'em coming!"

Finally, the boys are done. Gwen has not touched her steak. I've finished my chicken but have no memory of eating it. We get the check. Including the tip, it's the most expensive meal Gwen and I have ever eaten out. And we're nauseated from the stress.

The moral of the story? *Don't skip lunch*. I'm serious. I firmly believe the world would be two steps closer to peace if everyone, especially children, could eat a proper lunch every single day.

Chapter 41

Choosing a School

Noah is ready for first grade. There's no question where he will go to school. That would be like asking the Amish whether little Yoder will attend the new technology magnet school in the city or the local one-room schoolhouse.

In Northampton, Massachusetts, if you are embarrassed to own a computer and if you have convinced yourself that sugar and television are as much a national problem as the budget deficit, then you send your kids to the Waldorf school.

This means that Noah will learn to knit before he learns to read. It means that I have two, maybe three, more years of being better than him at drawing, painting, identifying the instruments in a symphony, and caring for livestock. It means that very soon, he will be, in general, a better, more well-rounded person than his dad.

Last week I sat in on Noah's class during parents' day. The children said hello to the teacher and then to us. They started in a circle and played games that develop coordination, rhythm, timing, and social skills. Then they went to their desks to work on the letter *M*. They learn to write it properly. I guarantee that any Waldorf student has better penmanship than you. Afterward, they sat, mesmerized, as their teacher told the story of Jack and the Beanstalk. He did not read from a book, but orated.

I want to convince Noah's teacher to present all this in a workshop at Kripalu. It would be a Waldorf version of the movie *Billy Madison* — we'd do a six-day workshop, one day devoted to each grade. Monday you're in first grade working on rhythm and hand-eye coordination, Tuesday you're in second, and so on. Maybe I could finally get some rhythm and learn to dance. This sort of education would have saved me twenty years of trying to connect my head to my body.

Every morning I drop Noah off at school. We park in the gravel drive. We walk past the breathtaking views of Mount Holyoke Range. Past the cows. Past the donkey and the goats. We break into a race. I am the color commentator, "Dad is in the lead. It's sure to be his day! Yes, Dad is ahead by two backpacks. Wait, what's this? Noah is gaining! Noah is closing in. Oh. My. Goodness. It's Noah Leaf! Noah Leaf WINS!"

During the race we veer to avoid two chickens pecking at the ground. We enter the building. It smells of soup. Homemade, from organic veggies grown by the children. Noah's cubby overflows with knitting projects, collected sticks and rocks, a felted bag containing a change of clothes, and his indoor shoes, into which he will change, Mr. Rogers–like, each morning.

Benji is in Waldorf for nursery school. His classroom is pure sweetness. A bin of silk scarves in warm pastels. A wooden play kitchen. Wooden blocks of every shape and size. A sand table. Handmade dolls. Not a single squeaking, buzzing, or talking toy in the room. And heavens to Betsy, no plastic.

During outdoor playtime, the children play amid the clucking chickens come snow, sleet, or driving rain. Waldorf nursery and kindergarten education encourages imaginative play. One day at the end of my workday, I receive a text from Gwen: "Get ice cream. Vanilla." I get home, and Benji has been inconsolable looking for his ice cream from school. We can't imagine what is up. I doubt ice cream has even crossed the nursery classroom's threshold. The school does not even allow refined sugar.

And then we figure it out. One of the children had started an ice cream store during playtime, and Benji had "purchased" a cone (a stick from the play yard). He had brought it home but left it in the car. Gwen didn't realize, because to her it looked exactly like every other stick that sits on the floor below Benji's seat. Once she got it for him, he was happy as could be and pretended to lick the imaginary cone.

In my first experience of Waldorf schools, twenty years ago, I worked in an afterschool program at a Waldorf school in New Jersey. During my first day on the job, a first-grader taught me to knit, played me a song on the recorder, and looked at me like an alien when I was afraid to touch a chicken. "Like this," she said, as she scooped up the chicken and gathered the day's egg.

A friend of ours took her son out of the school. She felt it was too perfect. Too sheltered and privileged. Another friend fears that in ten years his daughter will do a lot of cocaine in college after the shock of leaving utopia.

If you go in for this sort of farmish, artsy, peace–love–and–brown rice lifestyle, then it really is utopia. Though, I must admit that, unfortunately, it does feel a bit privileged. After all, even with partial financial aid, who can afford to pay for elementary school? In my estimation, there are basically two camps. There are those who, like my family, get help from grandparents to afford the tuition. And there are those whom you are sure must have hit it very big in the tech boom of the late '90s. Now, these folks generally live in straw-bale yurts built on thirty-seven acres of land.

I know that many folks who would like to send their kids to

Waldorf simply can't do it, so every day I am grateful to my parents for helping out. I like to think of the tuition as tithing at a church or synagogue. Really, that's what the school is to us.

Rudolf Steiner, the founder of Waldorf Schools, believed that each human being is born with a calling, a unique mission. A karmic purpose. The aim of the school is to foster the unfolding of that purpose and to provide the tools for each child to grow up pursuing his or her heartfelt calling, be it for music, mathematics, medicine, construction, farming, or philosophy.

Designing and founding this school and its pedagogy would be enough to be anyone's crowning lifetime achievement. An exceptional person's singular gift to the world. But not this guy. To Steiner, it was a day's work. Besides founding the Waldorf schools, he coined a philosophy, developed a system of medicine, designed buildings, and invented biodynamic farming.

Until doing research for this book, I knew almost nothing about Steiner and the underlying Waldorf philosophies. Turns out ol' Rudy was a nutter, first-class. Which is great. I mean, who in history who has made a difference wasn't?

Steiner makes the rest of us look like Muggles. He gained his knowledge of farming, education, politics, architecture, and art from meditation and astral projection. He would sit and contemplate a thing and in so doing he would open up to its truth, its history, its future. He would transcend the material world and see the world of spirit.

Pretty groovy, that's for sure.

You probably did not know this about Steiner because he is always depicted in a starched collar, tie, and dark suit, which make him look conservative, like any other top intellectual. But these were simply standard raiment, even for a hippie, in 1900. Today he'd be clad in ripped jeans, a Mexican serape, and John Lennon glasses.

And he'd be hanging out in New Age stores that sell incense and angels cards.

But that's just the point. When did spirit leave the mainstream? When did soul become marginalized? I'd like to see Steiner and Waldorf education in the mainstream, right in PS 101 or at my old elementary school in New Jersey. After all, Steiner created the very first Waldorf school at the request of the Waldorf-Astoria Cigarette Company for their employees' children. Does it get any more conventional than that?

In the words of His Holiness the Dalai Lama, "It is vital that when educating our children's brains that we do not neglect to educate their hearts."

Chapter 42

Free-Range Parenting

*W*hat if you lose your son for a minute in the mall? Will he be snapped up by a deviant with yellow teeth and a Def Leppard T-shirt?

Lenore Skenazy, author of *Free-Range Kids*, says, "Absolutely not."

Skenazy is hell-bent on showing parents that the world is not as unsafe as they think. Her self-proclaimed cause: "Fighting the belief that our children are in constant danger from creeps, kidnapping, germs, grades, flashers…baby snatchers, bugs, bullies, men, sleepovers and/or the perils of a nonorganic grape."

I disagree with her about the nonorganic grape. But otherwise, I'm on board. Noah is seven years old and seeking more independence, so I could use a dose of her antianxiety medicine.

Skenazy wants us to stop being helicopter parents. She wants us to let kids play outside, experiment, and be more independent. This, she posits, makes them happier, smarter, and more empowered.

In the Netherlands, reports Skenazy, four-year-olds romp around the playground unattended. In Lithuania, parents still leave their babies in strollers outside the market while they shop. And in lots of places around Europe, little kids ride their bicycles to school. This is true. My friend Yolanthe, who has moved to the Netherlands, confirms, "Yes, kids start riding at age four so they can bike to school by five."

Skenazy notes that when we hover over our kids to protect them, kids get the message that they're helpless without us. So what should we do? Says Skenazy, "Train our kids to look both ways, wash their hands, and never go off with strangers," and then give them some freedom.

To ease our collective anxiety, Skenazy gives facts and figures to debunk some of the most prevalent parenting fears. Here are a few that caught my attention:

1. *Germs.* Skenazy points out that if noted germophobe Howard Hughes lived today, he might not seem quite so loony. These days pumping hand sanitizer, swabbing surfaces with antibacterial wipes, and bringing your own place mats to restaurants are perfectly acceptable.

   Skenazy describes the "hygiene hypothesis," the notion that excessive hygiene actually leads to a weaker immune system and is associated with problems such as asthma and allergies. She cites a 1999 study that compared kids who were regularly exposed to cow dung (i.e., who grew up on farms) to those who, not so much. The study found that farm kids had half the incidences of asthma. Conclusion: Allowing children's immune systems to do some push-ups builds muscles for a lifetime. Please note: Do not smear cow dung on your children. Their young immune systems will get a very fine workout if you just allow them to play outside and dig in the dirt.

2. *Stranger danger.* Skenazy notes that strangers are not the problem. In fact, they can be the solution. Kids need to know that if there is a problem, strangers are exactly who they can reach out to. In the immeasurably unlikely event that someone approaches your bicycling children and tells them to get in the van, kids should be prepared. Skenazy recommends teaching kids to throw out their hands in the symbol for "stop," to scream for help so anyone nearby can hear, and to run or ride off like hell. The motto, says Skenazy, should not be "Don't talk to strangers"; it should be "Don't go off with strangers."

3. *Halloween.* Skenazy wants us to reclaim Halloween. She wants kids to trick-or-treat without parents, she wants folks to give out home-baked cookies and brownies, and she wants to get caramel apples, candy apples, and plain old apples back into the mix. So she looked into the number of Halloween poisonings and deaths.

   Skenazy found a hospital in Columbus, Ohio, that offers free X-rays of Halloween candy for concerned parents. The good news? The hospital has *never* found anything questionable. Which makes sense for Ohio. But what about elsewhere in the country? My home state of New Jersey, for example? Skenazy looked into the number of incidents of Halloween candy poisoning across the United States. Guess what she found.

   One hundred?

   One thousand!?

   Oh, my! Save us! Certainly not four thousand?!

   Nope. Zero. A big doughnut. Joel Best, professor of sociology and criminal justice at the University of Delaware, studied crime reports dating back to 1958 and found zero recorded incidents of trick-or-treaters being injured or dying from apples with razor blades or poisoned Halloween candy.

4.   *Eating raw cookie dough.* Everyone knows to avoid raw eggs. And since raw cookie dough contains this lethal killer, I would no sooner eat raw cookie dough than I would drink raw sewage. I am appalled that Ben & Jerry's still offers it (even eggless) as a flavor.

   But what did Skenazy find?

   According to a 2002 US Department of Agriculture study, 0.003 percent of the sixty-nine billion eggs produced each year carry salmonella. That's one is thirty thousand. And what if you eat the unlucky one? Well, then you still have a 94 percent chance of never even needing to see a doctor. You might have a bellyache, but no big deal.

   What's the worst-case scenario? You could die. And the chances of that? Skenazy says about one in fifty million. Which is about fifty times *less* than your chances of being struck by lightning this year.

5.   *Warm tuna sandwiches.* I loved tuna sandwiches when I was a boy. I can vividly recall opening the baggie and taking out the smelly, warm sandwich, mayo dripping, bread soggy. Yet now I would never eat warm mayo, let alone serve it to my boys. My sister and I call each other weekly to ask, "I have turkey that's been in the fridge for three days. Is it still good?"

   Skenazy tells us that we don't need, and have never needed, our insulated bags and cute SpongeBob ice packs to keep our kids' tuna cold. Mayonnaise, she says, is made with vinegar and helps tuna keep.

Hmm. Not so sure about this one. In fact, kids in my school threw up all the time. My elementary school was a vomit fest. It was like a frat party. I have many vivid memories of our janitor, Uncle Rex, coming in to clean it up. He had a powder he'd sprinkle on the puke to dry it up. Then he'd sweep it into a dustbin.

Skenazy may be right on this one, but for now, I'm sticking with ice packs and insulated lunch pails.

6. *Eating snow*. Snow was a staple of childhood in times of yore. But has it become hazardous? Skenazy's findings: No way. As long as it's not yellow. The study that caused a stir a few years ago, leading to headlines such as "Study Warns against Snow," says Skenazy, had nothing to do with eating it. The study pointed out that when snow forms it can cling to bacteria that cause disease in tomato and green bean plants. But nothing about disease in humans. So unless you are a tomato or green bean, says Skenazy, snow is perfectly safe. Eat up.

7. *Being dragged off by a wild animal*. What's the chance of this happening? For my boys it seems pretty high. I live in bear country. Last summer, a bear stopped in the backyard for a dip in Noah and Benji's plastic kiddie pool. Thankfully, they were not in it. We also have coyotes, deer, and some very fierce-looking bunnies. So the boys being dragged off by a wild animal is something I think about. And unfortunately, Noah seems to have caught on to the fact that I think about it. I think this is how we pick up our phobias, from our parents. If they are afraid, something must truly be amiss.

But Skenazy indicates that the number of children mauled by wild animals while in the safety of their backyards is nearly zero. That's right. Almost none. According to Skenazy this sort of thing pretty much happens only to negligent circus performers and zookeepers.

I was uncomfortable with that last one, so I checked, and a study published in 2004 by the University of California, Davis, documents thirty-five instances in California between 1978 and 2003 of children being attacked or dragged off by a coyote. Granted, every one of these thirty-five was rescued by a parent or neighbor. But, still, they were bitten and dragged off.

So, again, I think I need to ignore Skenazy on this one and continue to keep an eye on my kids in the backyard. At least until they weigh thirty pounds and are bigger than your average coyote.

Which makes me question her raw egg and her tuna hypotheses even more. In fact, you know what? I'm starting to think that Skenazy would not like me very much. My book with its cosleeping and cloth diapers and Playful Parenting probably seems pretty neurotic to her. Plus, we disagree about the tuna and the coyotes.

So I'm going to continue washing my hands after I crack eggs, and I'll keep my tuna salad in the fridge. I called my sister just this morning about some leftover bacon.

But even so, Skenazy has changed me. There is no doubt that kids need more free time and more play outside. And that empowering kids with appropriate levels of independence makes them stronger and more self-confident. After all, if we never remove the training wheels and don't let go of the bike, our children can never learn to ride.

So even amid my reservations, I've found myself going free-range. Just last week I asked Noah to venture a few aisles away from me in the supermarket to pick out fruit. And yesterday, when Noah and I were supposed to go for a bicycle ride together but I needed to stay home with Benji, I found myself saying, "Go ahead, sweetie.

You can ride by yourself down the road to Marc Circle (a cul-de-sac) and do some loops."

Noah was thrilled. He tore off down the street. He gathered speed, neared Marc Circle, started turning, took it a bit too wide, hit his tire on the curb, flipped off his bicycle, hit his bike helmet against the pavement, rolled two times, and cried.

I jogged to him.

He could stand.

I patted him down. Bloody scrapes on his knees and right elbow, but nothing serious.

I carried him home.

We are suing Skenazy.

Obviously.

But the experiment was actually a massive success. Noah stood proudly as Gwen washed his knees and elbow. Proud not of his cuts but of his independence. Proud of his short mission. And happy, I think, that I believed in him. That I trusted him. If I trust him, well then, he figures, he must be pretty great.

Maybe kids are not as breakable as I thought. Could it be that my anxieties about falling from a bicycle and eating spoiled eggs and falling from a trampoline are more dangerous than a scrape, occasional bellyache, or even twisted ankle? Maybe fearing nature is actually more harmful to health than an occasional bee sting? Maybe as I come to realize how strong Noah and Benji are, they will believe it too.

And maybe, just maybe, as I come to see that strangers are not in fact incompetent, evil, and plotting but are, instead, competent, kindly, and trustworthy, perhaps I will finally accept that so, too, am I.

Chapter 43

CTFD

I've been attempting to study and apply the best holistic parenting advice I can find. I've immersed myself in cosleeping and cloth diapers, and I've tried Attachment, Unconditional, Playful, Simplicity, and Free-Range Parenting.

I assess these approaches through the lens of consciousness. I won't follow a dogma. I want something that asks me to be more conscious. More empowered. More alert to my feelings. More present with my boys.

The good doctors Sears and Spock tell me that with tiny babies, I already know just what to do. I need only tap into my instincts. Sure, it doesn't hurt to Google the proper swaddling technique or to take a tip for the best brand of baby carrier, but for the big stuff, like how to nurture my children, I already know best.

Alfie Kohn and Adele Faber provide invaluable tools for surfing the wild seas of the post-toddler years. Essentially *How to Talk So Kids Will Listen & Listen So Kids Will Talk*. That about sums it up. Alfie tells me that the relationship matters most, that I need to get conscious and respond not from habit but directly to each moment.

And to ensure that my boys feel loved for who they are, not for what they do.

Next, Payne and Skenazy give me possibly the most crucial advice, especially as kids get a tad older: Back off. Don't hover or micromanage. Be a loving, reliable, ready resource, but don't jump in and take over at the first sign of challenge or struggle.

This makes sense to me; if there's one thing my yoga and meditation practice has shown me it is that happy is not the opposite of sad. Happiness is the result of fully experiencing myself and my feelings. Of allowing myself to experience the depth of a feeling, even of sadness.

When we allow kids their independence and empower them to have their own experiences, they learn to trust themselves. They develop fortitude and courage and realize that's it safe to have emotions and to see a feeling through.

This hands-on, hands-off approach is captured beautifully by Skenazy and Payne, and perhaps equally effectively, if less gracefully, by Dad blogger David Vienna in his CTFD approach, which stands for "calm the fuck down." According to Vienna, when you are worried that you are not imparting enough wisdom to your children or that your son's friend has already learned to read, just follow these simple steps:

1.   Calm the fuck down.
2.   There is no second step.

Make no mistake. I don't have it all figured out. I'm about as neurotic as the next guy. Maybe just a bit more. And that's why I know that another sure key to parenting is patience, compassion, forgiveness, and even faith, in my kids, of course, but also in myself. To follow my heart and push myself and take risks and try my very hardest and then to forgive myself and try again. And, really, to trust that my best is actually probably just fine. This not only keeps me off the bottle but provides a model for my boys. If I forgive myself, if I love myself unconditionally for who I am rather than for what I do, I have a very strong hunch that Noah and Benji will learn to do exactly the same for themselves.

And, really, what else could I possibly hope for? This is the very aim, I'd say, of parenting. The reason we do all that we do. So it almost feels like cheating. It's like a back door through a computer's firewall. We just hacked the system. If, with humility, we forgive and accept and love ourselves, unconditionally, then our kids will forgive and accept and love themselves, unconditionally.

And I'm pretty sure that would be pretty darn great.

Epilogue

Be Loved

It is a bit embarrassing to have been concerned with the human problem all one's life and find at the end that one has no more to offer by way of advice than, "Try to be a little kinder."

— Aldous Huxley

I'm finally reading *The Continuum Concept* by Jean Liedloff. I've heard a lot about this book, and going in, I already know several things. I know that it's one of those tough parenting reads. The kind of book that when you're done, you find yourself in the fetal position, rocking for comfort. The kind of book that makes you want to shake your fist at the government, phone your mom to cry, and call your kids to beg their forgiveness.

In the book, Liedloff relates her adventures in the jungles of South America, where she lived with the Ye'kuana people, who were relatively untouched by our society. Apart from having smartphones. Okay, no smartphones, but they did cheat a little by replacing their homemade stone machetes with metal ones. Besides that, they were untouched. And while hanging out with the Ye'kuana, Liedloff noticed that they were happy, that they enjoyed themselves no matter what they were doing, and, get this, that they didn't belittle and mock one another. This was no episode of HBO's *Entourage* in the Venezuelan jungle.

Liedloff traced the Ye'kuana's jolly temperaments back to their parenting. In particular, the women would wear their babies in slings and wraps with skin-to-skin contact as they performed their daily habits of gathering and preparing food. They did not pressure the babes to sit on their own by 5.2 months, and they did not plunk them in front of *Baby Einstein* videos. In fact, they held their children from the moment they were born until they could crawl away.

And their children prospered. They were part of society. They helped out as soon as they were old enough. They did not seem to experience teen angst or say things like, "I hate you, Mom!" And at turning twenty, they did not dye their hair purple and move to the East Village.

Sounds great, but when I finished Liedloff's book, as expected, I wanted to find a tall Venezuelan waterfall and jump to my demise. Because, according to Liedloff, the fact that we were not held continuously, and I mean 24/7, as babies explains why we don't feel safe in the womb of the world. It explains why we feel unloved and unworthy of love. It explains our depression, anxiety, and anger. It explains why my emotions seem to run the small interval between Woody Allen and George Costanza.

Perhaps this is the fault of a society that doesn't require employers to offer longer maternity leaves. Or of a weak economy that necessitates that both parents make a living. Or maybe it's the result of our discomfort with showing affection that dates back to Queen Victoria. Personally, I still like to blame George W. Bush. Pretty much for anything.

Either way, what can we do about it?

Well, according to Liedloff, first of all, if you have a baby, hold it and sleep with it, and carry it in a sling while you do your daily chores. The best bet would be to gather roots and berries and fetch water and grind corn. If that's inconvenient, just do your work and do the dishes and cook and clean, but hold your baby all along. Unless your work involves driving a truck. In that case, make other arrangements for your baby. Or consider moving to Canada. Canada is a world leader in maternity leave, at an average of fifty weeks.

And don't judge or have expectations of the little tyke. Let your babe have his or her own unique experience.

And, perhaps most important, tap into and follow your own intuition. Don't follow in the footsteps of the Ye'kuana; seek what they sought. Human beings, like all animals, have evolved for millions of years to know *exactly* how to parent their young. And you know how too.

But here's the trickiest part. What do we do for ourselves? How can we heal our own inner George Costanza? I was depressed about this...until I hatched a plan. I decided that it was not too late for me to reclaim a feeling of safety and love in the world.

I call this my Be Loved experiment, and I've been practicing now for, like, three months.

In the first version of this experiment, I would sit on my meditation cushion and visualize everyone I know standing in line and, one by one, giving me a hug. I was like the selfish opposite of Amma, the hugging saint. This was a high, to be sure. But then I'd leave my cushion and be appalled at how crude and unkind people could be. In my visualizations, I was receiving gooey, unconditional love, but in real life, when people were not the doting lovers of my meditation, I felt judged, hurt, and rejected.

When I told this to Edmund, my osteopathic shaman, he shook his head. It's unwise to pray to the living. So I switched and went right to the top, to the all-mother. To the Elvis of unconditional lovers. To God. Now I'd visualize God hugging me. I'd sink into her and feel her enveloping me. I'd imagine her wearing me in a giant wrap; she'd play with my toes and kiss my head.

This was nice. I was reclaiming the continuum and feeling loved. But God can be difficult to visualize, so now I think of my grandma. I remember cuddling on her lap. I visualize her hugging me. I sink into her, and she envelops me.

I practice every day. I practice being loved and letting love in. In the words of the thirteenth-century Persian poet Jalāl ad-Dīn Muhammad Rūmī, a sure favorite with yogis on Facebook, "Your task is not to seek for love, but merely to seek and find all the barriers within yourself that you have built against it."

Some days are better than others. Some days I feel adrift. And other days, and there are more and more of these as I practice, I'm surprised, not by how unkind people can be, but by how connected and loved I feel.

I'm working on this. I know that it's important work. I think it may well be the very key to parenting and yoga alike. I know that when I feel loved, I am a better parent. My worst parenting moments, heck, my worst moments in general, stem from feeling unloved. That's when I am greedy, unkind, or apathetic. But when I feel fully loved, I can love Gwen and my boys fully. When I feel fully loved I can love and accept each moment in all its gritty glory. I can see more clearly and be more conscious. I can more easily access my intuition and instincts. When I feel fully loved, I can love fully. Period. And that's all I really want to do.

Acknowledgments

That's going in the book!

— Brian Leaf

*H*ats off to Gwen. Let's face it, having one's husband write a memoir must be somewhat concerning. And a parenting memoir must be all the worse. But Gwen has been nothing but enthusiastic and supportive. And if she's supportive and patient with me, imagine how she is with our children. Noah, Benji, and I are three very lucky boys. We are truly blessed, and I am forever grateful. Gwen, I love you. Immeasurably.

Also a huge gracias to my editor at New World Library, Jason Gardner, for championing the book and for a fantastic edit. He's the one who first came up with the idea for the *It Gets Better* videos for new parents. Much needed, I think. Plus, he really saved the project. Without his suggested changes to the manuscript, you surely would have flung this book across the room against the wall many pages ago.

Thanks to all the terrific people at New World Library: Kim Corbin, the ultimate publicist, for reminding me to smile and skip (check out her website at www.iskip.com), Munro Magruder for selling the heck out of the book, Tracy Cunningham for her gorgeous design, Mimi Kusch for her genius edits, and Marc Allen and Shakti Gawain for starting it all.

Thanks to my sister and brother, Julie and Larry Leaf. I am blessed to never have known what it is to feel alone in the world.

Thanks to my wonderful community of friends at Kripalu, the Hartsbrook School, Rocky Hill Cohousing, birthing class, my Thursday writers' group, Gwen's prenatal yoga class, the Cooley baby group, and Mothering.com, as well as to Matthew Andrews and Matt Oestreicher for sharing the journey.

Thanks oodles to Noah and Benji. These guys make Unconditional Parenting easy. Noah and Benji, I relish every day that I get to be your dad.

Thanks to my mom and dad, Susan and Manny Leaf, for teaching me, by your gracious example, how to love. There is no higher path.

My dad, Manny Leaf, died on March 14, 2013. He came to the United States at age eleven. He built his business. He loved his family. He was a beautiful soul. He may well have been a saint, at least in my eyes. I love you, Dad.

And finally, my sincerest apologies to Ed, the psychotherapist in town whom I used to judge. I'd see him walking around downtown disheveled, spacey, and always in a rush. Ed, I knew you had a newborn, but back then, before I had children of my own, I simply had no idea what that really meant. I owe you a lunch.

Appendix

Ayurvedic Constitutional Survey and Recommendations

*F*ill out the following Ayurvedic constitutional questionnaire. For each row, circle characteristics in the one or two columns that best describe you for that trait.

	VATA	PITTA	KAPHA
BONE STRUCTURE	thin, slight	moderate	broad
BODY WEIGHT	difficult to gain	moderate	easy to gain
SKIN	dry, cool, dark	soft, oily, warm, fair	thick, oily, cool, pale
HAIR	black, dry, kinky	soft, oily, yellow, early gray, red	thick, oily, wavy
APPETITE	variable	strong	slow, but steady

	VATA	PITTA	KAPHA
THIRST	variable	strong	low
MIND	active, restless	aggressive, sharp	calm, slow
EMOTIONAL TEMPERA- MENT UNDER STRESS	fearful, insecure, unpredictable	aggressive, irritable	calm, greedy, attached
RESOLVE	changeable	fanatic	steady
MEMORY	recent good, long term poor	sharp	slow, but prolonged
DREAMS	fearful, movement	fire, anger, violence	watery, romantic
SLEEP	interrupted	little but sound	heavy, prolonged
SPEECH	fast	sharp, cutting	slow

Adapted from Vasant Lad, *Ayurveda: The Science of Self Healing: A Practical Guide* (Lotus Press, 1984).

The sum of the checks down each column indicates the number for *vata*, *pitta*, and *kapha*. If one of these numbers is much larger than each of the others, such as 11 *vata*, 4 *pitta*, and 3 *kapha*, then that *dosha* is the one to watch for imbalances.

If the survey shows a predominance of *vata*:

1. Keep warm, and wear soft, comfortable clothing. Make your bed into a soft, comfy haven.
2. Eat mostly cooked foods and use a bit of spice. Eat at a table, in a relaxed setting, not on the go or standing at the sink.
3. Keep a regular routine, and look over your schedule at the beginning of each day, so your mind can relax and know what's coming.
4. Practice gentle forms of exercise.
5. Spend quiet time in nature, ideally near a lake or gently flowing stream. Sit under a tree.
6. Avoid or cut back on caffeine, wheat, sugar, and processed foods.

If the survey shows a predominance of *pitta*:

1. Keep cool. Get lots of fresh air, but avoid too much direct sun. Take evening walks in the moonlight. The moon is very soothing to *pitta*.
2. Eat lots of fresh fruits and vegetables.
3. Avoid very spicy, very salty, and very oily foods.
4. Watch your tendency toward perfectionism, competition, and intensity. Bring in softness and love.
5. Express your feelings in constructive ways. Be gentle on yourself and others.
6. Avoid or cut back on caffeine, wheat, sugar, and processed foods.

If the survey shows a predominance of *kapha*:

1. Get lots of vigorous exercise, every day.
2. Avoid fatty and fried foods. Eat lots of veggies, and cook with a bit of spice.
3. Eat less bread.
4. Avoid getting into a rut. Try new things, take challenges, travel.
5. Practice expressing your voice and your feelings, and spend some time creating every day. Draw, paint, sculpt, sing, dance, play an instrument, imagine.
6. Avoid or dramatically cut back on wheat, sugar, and processed foods.

Reading Group Guide

1. In the preface, Brian proves he's a parent by writing, "Inside my coat pocket right now are one diaper (clean), one pair of children's underwear (soiled), one unscratched lottery ticket, and countless teething biscuit and rice cake crumbs." What's your proof?

2. Regarding his wedding, Brian states, "I had always wondered how I could one day have a wedding that would reflect my eclectic spiritual beliefs but not alienate my Jewish relatives from New Jersey. I needed a druid, a rabbi, and a swami to co-officiate." Were there family or friends that you took into account when planning your wedding? Did you appease them?

3. Brian and Gwen decided to tell family and friends they were pregnant during the first trimester based on a friend's advice: "Why wait? Tell people that you'd want to know if you were to lose the baby. You'd need

their love and support. Why be isolated and alone?" At what point in the pregnancy would you share the news?

4.   When Brian asked one of the midwives, "What do husbands usually do during labor?" she answered, "You know, they usually eat an egg salad sandwich and watch the game in the TV room." Does this seem fair to you? Does it match your experience?

5.   In chapter 33, Brian describes the process he and Gwen used to arrive at their children's names. How did you or would you choose names?

6.   Brian's final comment on circumcision: "Ironically, for me, the decision actually did come down to God. I trust her, and I don't think she designed the human body with a throwaway foreskin, like an Old Navy tag we're supposed to remove before wearing. I think the human body is holy and magical and perfect as is." What's your opinion? Would you choose circumcision?

7.   In a chart on page 46, Brian offers three categories of parents, *mainstream*, *alternative*, and *nearly Amish*. He places himself somewhere between *alternative* and *nearly Amish*. Where do you fit on the chart?

8.   One possible criticism of the book is Brian's use of humor when discussing very important and even controversial topics. Do you appreciate his use of humor? Does it make the material accessible? Does it add to or dilute the discussion of the issues?

9. In chapter 11, Brian lays out Dr. Sears's seven Bs of Attachment Parenting:

   Birth bonding
   Read and respond to your baby's cues, that is, cries
   Breastfeeding
   Babywearing (carry baby in a sling or carrier)
   Bedding close to baby (cosleeping)
   Balance and boundaries
   Beware of baby trainers

   How do the seven Bs sit with you? Do you practice Attachment Parenting?

10. Regarding number 6 (Balance and boundaries) on Dr. Sears's list, Brian explains, "Take care of yourself. Put on your own oxygen mask first, as they say. A healthy baby needs a healthy mom and dad.

    Take a night off. Hire a sitter, or call Grandma. Exercise. Eat well. You'll be a better parent when (at least a few of) your own needs are met." If you are a parent, how's this going for you? Do you take care of yourself?

11. In chapter 12, Brian describes his family's sleeping arrangement. Did you have any reaction to this? What arrangement do you use?

12. Early in the book, Brian says he and Gwen used cloth diapers and sometimes disposables. Later Brian discusses elimination communication. What was your diapering choice? Why?

13. In chapter 12, Brian sees an osteopathic shaman after Gwen kicked him in the nose as they rescued Noah

from behind the couch. Do you have any kid-induced injury stories?

14. In chapter 17, Brian apologizes to Noah for holding him down while the optometrist put drops in Noah's eyes. Do you think Brian was right to apologize? Can you recall a time when you apologized or wanted to apologize to your kids?

15. Brian briefly describes the work of B. F. Skinner and his influence on education and parenting: "Skinner demonstrated that a rat who gets a treat from pressing a lever will repeatedly press the lever. He then extended this finding to humans, espousing 'operant conditioning' in raising children, that is, using rewards and punishments to elicit desired behavior." What Skinner influences can you find in schools, parenting advice, and society in general?

16. Regarding elimination communication, discussed in chapter 26, Brian quips, "It seems just, well, barbaric. Which it is, and let's face it, that's a good thing. The opposite, being civilized, comes with all kinds of problems." What do you think he means by this? Do you agree?

17. In the Eric Carle Museum, described on page 130, amid a crowded hallway of parents and children Brian's son shouts that he wants to see Brian's "hairyyy peeeeeniiiiis." What's you most embarrassing parenting story?

18. What do you think of Brian's description of Playful Parenting in chapter 30? Would you try any of Cohen's recommendations with your own family?

19. Brian summarizes Adele Faber and Elaine Mazlish's model from *How to Talk So Kids Will Listen & Listen So Kids Will Talk* as follows:

    When your kids speak, listen with full attention.
    Rather than responding with questions and advice, acknowledge your child's feelings with, "Oh...mmm... I see."
    Give your child's feeling a name.

    Have you tried this with your own children?

20. Had you already heard of Simplicity Parenting? Brian quotes Kim John Payne, author of *Simplicity Parenting*: "The great news is that we don't have to do that much to introduce our kids to the benefits of their own intelligence and freedom. Just relax a little bit. Give them just a bit more space than you think you can." Does giving them more space scare you? Does it appeal to you, as well? If so, how would you give your children more space than you think you can?

21. Brian writes a lot about listening to his parenting instincts. He writes, "Sure, it doesn't hurt to Google the proper swaddling technique or to take a tip for the best brand of baby carrier, but for the big stuff, like how to nurture my children, I already know best." Do you agree? Do you try to listen for and act from instinct?

22. What do you think Brian means by Conscious Parenting?

23. What is a parenting yogi? Are you such a person?

About the Author

*B*rian Leaf is the director of the New Leaf Learning Center and the author of twelve books, including *Misadventures of a Garden State Yogi*. His work has been featured in *Yoga Journal*, *Yoga International*, *USA TODAY*, and *The Huffington Post*, and he blogs for Mothering.com and Kripalu.org. Visit Brian at his website, www.Misadventures-of-a-Yogi.com.

NEW WORLD LIBRARY is dedicated to publishing books and other media that inspire and challenge us to improve the quality of our lives and the world.

We are a socially and environmentally aware company. We recognize that we have an ethical responsibility to our customers, our staff members, and our planet.

We serve our customers by creating the finest publications possible on personal growth, creativity, spirituality, wellness, and other areas of emerging importance. We serve New World Library employees with generous benefits, significant profit sharing, and constant encouragement to pursue their most expansive dreams.

As a member of the Green Press Initiative, we print an increasing number of books with soy-based ink on 100 percent postconsumer-waste recycled paper. Also, we power our offices with solar energy and contribute to non-profit organizations working to make the world a better place for us all.

Our products are available in bookstores everywhere.

www.newworldlibrary.com

At NewWorldLibrary.com you can download our catalog,
subscribe to our e-newsletter, read our blog,
and link to authors' websites, videos, and podcasts.

Find us on Facebook, follow us on Twitter, and watch us on YouTube.

Send your questions and comments our way!
You make it possible for us to do what we love to do.

Phone: 415-884-2100 or 800-972-6657
Catalog requests: Ext. 10 | Orders: Ext. 52 | Fax: 415-884-2199
escort@newworldlibrary.com

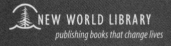 NEW WORLD LIBRARY
publishing books that change lives   14 Pamaron Way, Novato, CA 94949